The New Weight Loss Era:

Navigating Nutrition with a Dietitian's Expertise in the Age of Medications

KELLY SPRINGER, RD, MS, CDN

ACKNOWLEDGEMENTS

I am profoundly grateful to the dedicated team of professionals and students whose collective effort brought this book to fruition.

It is with immense appreciation that I acknowledge Shannon Hodson, a talented writer for Kelly's Choice, whose expertise and dedication were instrumental in transforming my Transformational Program into this book. Her meticulous attention to detail, coupled with two years of tireless work interviewing patients and adding supporting research, enriched this project immeasurably.

I extend my deepest gratitude to Cindy Debbold, my esteemed mentor, whose encouragement paved the way for the creation of the Transformational Program. Additionally, I am indebted to Dr. Margaret Voss and Dr. Kay Bruening, prestigious professors at Syracuse University, whose rigorous fact-checking and invaluable guidance ensured the accuracy and integrity of this manuscript.

Heartfelt thanks go to the students from the dietetics programs at Cornell University and Penn State University, whose collaboration in crafting the recipes added a nice dimension and value to the book.

I am very grateful for the many patients who welcomed the opportunity to have their case studies published in this book—only first names were used to protect our patients' privacy and confidentiality.

A special appreciation is reserved for Jourdan Garcia, talented photographer and head of marketing for Kelly's Choice; she photographed the recipes.

I express my gratitude to Abby Dean, RD, Kathryn Spychalski, RD, Jennifer Pacheco, and my mother, Peggy Lattimore, whose invaluable contributions during the editing process refined the content of this book.

Finally, my heartfelt thanks to my husband Greg, my daughters Ellie and Liv, my dedicated executive assistant, Clare Hoke, and all the exceptional employees at Kelly's Choice for their unwavering support and dedication.

ABOUT THE AUTHOR

A voice of authority and advocacy, Kelly Springer, RD, MS, CDN, is elevating the conversation around what it means to be truly healthy. Kelly founded Kelly's Choice in 2012 and has grown her business to the largest dietitian-owned nutritional consulting company in the world with over 50 talented dietitians who deliver exceptional precision nutrition services.

Kelly has been a keynote speaker and panelist at numerous conferences and workplaces across the globe, captivating audiences and inspiring them with her expertise and enthusiasm. Her impact extends to national television with features on Good Morning America, Fox 5 Atlanta, WCCO CBS Minneapolis, and many others. Kelly also serves as a spokesperson for exceptional health brands, elevating their profile through a variety of media platforms including television.

Kelly is a proud board member of the American Heart Association, advocating for heart health and wellness on a national level. She holds a bachelor's degree in nutrition from West Virginia University and a master's degree in health education from SUNY Cortland. Kelly's extensive experience includes serving as the division dietitian at Wegmans Food Markets and as a clinical dietitian at Auburn Hospital, specializing in bariatrics, critical care, and nutrition support. Learn more at kellyschoice.org.

CONTENTS

INTRODUCTION

I'm Kelly Springer, a registered dietitian and founder of Kelly's Choice, a company with amazing, dedicated registered dietitians like me. I am so glad you picked up this book!

I'm an enthusiastic health educator, mom, wife, pizza-holic and your supporter through this program. Kelly's Choice's tagline is "We are real people promoting real food." This is not a crazy fad diet; this is a lifestyle upgrade. This is a guide to help you lose weight and improve your quality of life. And if you are taking GLP-1 receptor agonists like Ozempic®, consider this book as a companion to your type-2 diabetes or weight-loss medication treatment.

GLP-1 receptor agonists have been on the market for quite some time, specifically prescribed and utilized to manage diabetes through improved blood glucose control. Over the years, we have witnessed firsthand how these medications not only help manage diabetes, but also support weight loss.

Recently, we have started seeing patients who are prescribed these medications based on obesity and associated risk factors alone. Our collective approach to these clients is to help them through their journey. At Kelly's Choice, we maintain a nonjudgmental policy and meet our patients where they are at. We are here to help our patients navigate any nutrition-related side-effects of GLP-1 receptor agonists, prevent potential nutrient deficiencies, promote gut health, and ensure adequate protein intake and hydration.

To sustain long-term weight loss, you should incorporate a multi-pronged approach and practice healthy habits consistently.

In a 2024 article published on the American Medical Association's website, Cardiologist Stephen Devries, MD, Executive Director of the educational nonprofit Gaples Institute in Chicago, and Harvard University professor, said: "If there's a chance of getting people off the (GLP-1 agonist receptor meds and maintaining weight loss, it will be important that they've established and maintained a healthy pattern of eating during the time they've been on the medication...For patients who do stay on the meds indefinitely, a high-quality diet will be crucial for optimal health and longevity."[i]

This book is a roadmap that will help you develop healthy habits you need in the areas of nutrition, exercise, and stress management.

Ultimately, throughout your journey, you will learn how to reduce your risk of chronic diseases, like heart disease and type-2 diabetes, and enhance your overall quality of life. And if you already have a chronic disease, you will improve the condition and may even be able to reverse it. As one patient, Vicky, has said to us recently, "You saved my life!"

If you think this program is going to have you counting calories and restricting yourself from your favorite foods, think again!

This is not about restriction; it's about satisfaction. You don't have to deny yourself a piece of cake at your daughter's birthday party. You can have that burger at your favorite burger joint on an occasional Saturday night. By following this program, you will improve your eating in such a way that these splurges will be possible and will not hold you back from achieving your health goals.

I don't label foods as "good" or "bad."

One Kelly's Choice dietitian, Jen, puts it this way: "The only foods that are 'bad' are foods that you are allergic to, recalled or rotten food, and fake food."

What Jen means by fake food is food with ingredients like silicone. What?! Yes, I found out that there was silicone in what I thought was a healthy avocado oil spray!

I prefer terms like healthier and better, than simply labeling foods as good or bad. It's all about choices and creating habits.

This program will empower you to invest in yourself and your overall wellness in the pursuit of living your best lives. A longer and happier life—something we all want, right?

Investing in yourself is the best investment you will ever make. When you invest in yourself, you will start to see a ripple effect in all aspects of your life. When you begin making small changes to your nutrition, you will not only improve your waistline, but you will also naturally improve your overall health.

It saddens me to know that approximately 6 in 10 adults are living with at least one chronic disease-some with two or more.[ii] The World Health Organization predicts that by 2030, approximately 70% of global deaths will be related to chronic disease. Chronic diseases such as heart disease, stroke, type-2 diabetes and obesity are driven by the epidemic of harmful lifestyle resulting from smoking, unhealthy diet, and physical inactivity.[iii] In 2016, 529,999 deaths (19.1% total deaths) were attributed to dietary risks.[iv]

By being here and reading this guide, you have already taken your first step to a healthier life. You should be proud of yourself! It's no easy feat, and seeking improvements and betterment is commendable. Making healthier choices and working to improve the quality of your diet can set you on the road to success.

Reducing body weight not only reduces your risk of chronic diseases, but proper nutrition can actually protect you from these diseases.

If you already have a chronic condition or disease, you might be thinking to yourself that it's too late. That doesn't always have to be the case. Weight loss and improved nutrition can help delay disease progression, reduce the risk of complications, and even reverse some diseases, like pre-diabetes and type-2 diabetes.

Take Michelle for example. She came to me in 2014 after being diagnosed with type-2 diabetes. She said to me, "My doctor said, 'Take this medicine, stop eating sweets, and here's your test kit.'"

While a prescription may improve your A1C, the tools in that toolbox are probably not enough to conquer chronic disease. Michelle was worried; though she was overweight, she thought she was healthy and was horrified when she researched the side effects of diabetes and learned that it could worsen her eyesight and her circulation, cause kidney disease, heart disease, and a whole slew of health problems. Fortunately, Michelle wanted guidance on how to change her eating. And that she did!

By implementing daily movement and slowly changing her meals, Michelle lost 110 pounds and reversed her type-2 diabetes. Her A1C no longer puts her in the diabetic or pre-diabetic category. She continues to maintain blood sugar levels within the normal range without taking medications to regulate them. She has maintained habits that she learned through this program, reduced her medication burden and associated costs, and still, ten years later, constantly thanks me for improving and extending her life!

What Michelle and all others value about this program is that it is educational; I am not here to just tell you what to eat, give you a meal plan, and send you on your way; I explain the why behind healthier choices, giving you knowledge and tools you can begin to rely on to make informed decisions. I will teach you how your body works and responds to different foods. This program is completely customizable to you and your lifestyle. Healthier choices can look different for everyone, depending on their schedule and responsibilities.

Whether you're a parent juggling the demands of a busy family schedule, a frequent traveler navigating airport dining options, a student managing academic commitments, or a professional with a hectic work life, this program is designed to seamlessly integrate into your routine.

I will filter through the confusing contradictions you hear about nutrition and find the answers for you!

My program has been utilized with over fifty worksites, dozens of schools, sports teams, and over one thousand private practice patients. The results have been amazing. I am all about population health and getting this education to everyone because *everyone* deserves to understand nutrition.

The food recommendations throughout this book may seem like those from the Mediterranean Diet, but here's the thing—the Mediterranean Diet is NOT a DIET; it's a LIFESTYLE. The Mediterranean Diet looks at some of the staples like whole grains, nuts, fruits, vegetables, fish, and olive oil consumed by Italians, Greeks, Egyptians, and others who live near the Mediterranean Sea; hundreds of research studies have shown that these food staples help with weight loss and help reduce the risk of heart disease. A 2020 metanalysis in the Critical Reviews of Food Science Nutrition examined many such studies and found that the Mediterranean Diet very effectively reduced the risk of heart disease and mortality for those who had heart disease as well as stroke and stroke-related mortality.[v]

Another study published in the Journal of the American Medical Association in 2018[vi] also revealed how powerful clean foods like those in the Mediterranean Diet could be in improving people's overall health. This $8 million trial by Stanford University researchers looked at 609 overweight adults for one year, placing some of those adults on a low-carb diet and some on a low-fat diet. While following these diets, both groups were given 22 lessons about making choices that were wholesome, low in sodium and added sugar, eating lots of vegetables and decreasing refined flour and processed foods.

While the intention of the study was to determine whether the low-fat or low-carb diet led to better outcomes, interestingly, the study found that both worked. And not because the foods were low-carb or low-fat, but because the study participants learned how to choose wholesome, less processed food!

The study participants in both groups lost an average of 12 pounds, and some lost more than 50 pounds. Additionally, they significantly improved their body fat percentage, waist size, blood pressure, and cholesterol and insulin levels, overall lowering their risk of diseases like type-2 diabetes, heart disease, and other serious chronic illnesses.

You might be wondering, what does this mean for me? Just like the Stanford University study, you will learn how to make informed choices on what nourishes your body and what doesn't. You can immediately start making changes that will have an impact on your nutrition and health. This is the foundation of this program.

The program starts off by delving into the mechanism of GLP-1 receptor agonists, so you have a better understanding of how the medication works. Then, we will introduce nutrition education and why it is important to develop healthy habits to create sustainable lifestyle changes.

In the second chapter you will read is about the Power of Five; these are the foods that fuel your body. The first one is carbohydrates. Yes, you read that right—this is *not* a grain-free diet; it is not low-carb either, but please don't be worried. You will learn why you need them (ahem, FIBER) and will be able to differentiate the carbs you should include in your daily diet and the ones to limit. The other foods in the Power of Five are protein, dairy, vegetables, and fruit. You will learn the importance of food synergy and how combining certain foods can help you balance your blood sugar levels and absorb powerful nutrients that will fight off invaders (known as free radicals) that are trying to inflame your body. Inflammation is responsible for weight gain and can be linked to almost all chronic conditions.

Balanced blood sugar is the most crucial element you need for an optimal lifestyle. While your GLP-1 receptor agonist can help with this, the power of nutritional strategies should not be overlooked.

For the next few chapters, we will dive into education about carbohydrates, protein, and fat, looking at how they function in your body and the best sources of each. There will also be a chapter fully dedicated to fruits and vegetables with strategies on how to effectively and deliciously incorporate them into your diet.

Once you have the foundational knowledge of the main food groups, you will learn skills on how to help maintain my suggestions with chapters dedicated to food shopping and meal planning as well as specifics about sugar and sodium. You will then learn about favorite meals and snacks...juicy secrets here!

Next, we get into improving lifestyle habits that will also support your health, like proper sleep, dining out healthfully, and eating mindfully.

We will tie everything together with a chapter on digestive health. A healthy gut is the foundation of a healthy body and mind.

Finally, I will educate you on how to maintain this lifestyle.

At the end of each chapter, you will have goals to accomplish in the areas of nutrition, hydration, and exercise before moving on to the next chapter.

Hydration is critical to combat some of the side effects that GLP-1s can cause, such as diarrhea.

Incorporating daily movement into your routine can facilitate weight loss and maintenance. Both cardiovascular exercise and strength training can contribute to calorie burning and improved metabolic health.

I highly encourage you to use a food diary, either a journal/notebook or an online platform.

There are some carefully curated recipes that are generally quick and easy to make provided at the end of the chapters and even more at the end of the book

Pace yourself through this process. Some people may be able to go through this in 12 weeks; for others it may take a year. And if you slip; don't stress. Life happens!

CHAPTER 1: THE COMBINATION OF NUTRITION EDUCATION AND GLP-1 RECEPTOR AGONISTS FOR WEIGHT LOSS SUCCESS

In the world of type-2 diabetes management and weight loss, GLP-1 (glucagon-like peptide-1 receptor agonists have emerged as game changers, offering a dual role in blood sugar regulation and appetite control. These medications, originally crafted for type-2 diabetes management, have captured attention for their ability to result in weight loss. Let's explore the mechanisms behind GLP-1 receptor agonists and uncover how they work in synergy with the power of nutrition.

GLP-1 receptor agonists include exenatide (Byetta®, Bydureon®), liraglutide (Victoza®, Saxenda®), dulaglutide (Trulicity®), semaglutide (Ozempic®), tirzepatide (Mounjaro®), and lixisenatide (Adlyxin®).

What are GLP-1s?

GLP-1 stands for glucagon-like peptide 1. It is naturally produced in the body, primarily in the intestines, in response to food intake. GLP-1 is a gut-derived peptide secreted from intestinal L-cells after a meal. GLP-1 receptors are found throughout the body including in the brain, gastrointestinal tract, the pancreas, and other organs. Its production serves several important physiological functions related to metabolism and digestion.

Here's why our bodies produce GLP-1

1) **Regulation of Insulin and Glucagon:** GLP-1 plays a crucial role in glucose metabolism. It stimulates the secretion of insulin from pancreatic beta cells while inhibiting the release of glucagon from pancreatic alpha cells. This dual action helps to regulate blood sugar levels by promoting glucose uptake into cells and suppressing the production of glucose by the liver.
2) **Appetite Regulation:** GLP-1 also plays a role in regulating appetite and food intake. It slows down gastric emptying, which helps to prolong the feeling of

fullness after a meal. This feeling results in reduced food intake, leading to weight loss.

3) **Cardiovascular Effects:** GLP-1 has been found to have cardiovascular benefits, including reducing blood pressure and improving cardiac function.

Particularly for people with type-2 diabetes, the body's natural production of GLP-1 has become insufficient or dysregulated. In such cases, pharmacological intervention with GLP-1 receptor agonists can help to restore balance and improve metabolic health[vii].

The pharmaceutical drugs known as GLP-1 receptor agonists work by mimicking the action of GLP-1 in the body. They bind to and activate the GLP-1 receptors on target cells, leading to similar effects. These drugs are used in the treatment of type-2 diabetes and obesity because they can improve blood sugar control, promote weight loss, and have potential cardiovascular benefits.

Semaglutide and Tirzepatide are the most popularly prescribed GLP-1 Receptor agonists.

Semaglutide is the active ingredient in Ozempic® and Wegovy®. It works as a GLP-1 receptor agonist to treat type-2 diabetes. Semaglutide is also used for weight loss.

Tirzepatide is the active ingredient in Mounjaro®, which can also treat type-2 diabetes and result in weight loss. Tirzepatide is a GLP-1 receptor agonist as well as a GIP (glucose-dependent insulinotropic polypeptide receptor agonist. GIP is another hormone your body makes after you eat.

The main difference between these two types of medications is that tirzepatide mimics two hormones while semaglutide mimics one.

How effective are GLP-1 Receptor Agonists?

GLP-1 receptor agonists are very effective at treating type-2 diabetes and weight-loss. Newly approved and emerging anti-obesity medications (AOMs can reduce body weight by about 15%, which has previously only been seen with bariatric surgeries and very low-calorie diets.[viii]

In the past 5 years, the number of patients with type-2 diabetes taking a GLP-1 medication has risen to 43%, and the number of patients diagnosed as overweight taking the medication has risen to 22%.

Nutrition Education: The Key Ingredient for Success

Enter nutrition education, the steadfast ally in the quest for sustained weight loss and overall health. It seems like common sense that once you stop taking a weight loss drug, the weight loss well, stops too. Weight gain is likely as well, potentially exceeding the weight that you started at. That is why nutrition education is a must-have companion when taking a GLP-1 receptor agonist. Here's how this dynamic duo collaborates:

Healthy Eating Habits: The foundation of success lies in embracing a diverse range of nourishing foods such as fruits, vegetables, lean proteins, and whole grains. Nutrition education takes center stage, empowering you to make informed choices that can support your health goals. GLP-1 receptor agonists can complement these efforts by promoting feelings of fullness, decreasing appetite and reducing intake. Some explain this as "quieting the food noise."

Regular Physical Activity: Registered Dietitians recognize that physical activity is essential for overall health and vitality. By incorporating regular exercise into your routine, you can enhance well-being and boost metabolism. Nutrition and exercise work hand in hand to promote a healthy lifestyle, with GLP-1 receptor agonists providing additional support by assisting with appetite control.

Behavioral Strategies: Addressing behaviors related to eating habits and emotional triggers is crucial for long-term success. Have you tried every diet on the market, and nothing worked? Nutrition education works best with behavior change to match. Registered Dietitians can help give you the knowledge and tools you need to make small, sustainable behavior modifications over time for lifelong success. GLP-1 receptor agonists can provide support in overcoming obstacles and fostering positive behavior change, acting as the catalyst for your health journey.

Commitment to Long-Term Health: Consistency is key in maintaining a healthy lifestyle. By practicing mindful eating, exercising regularly, and managing stress effectively, you can cultivate habits that promote lasting well-being.

Scientific studies also report the effectiveness of combining GLP-1 inhibitor therapy with nutrition intervention.

For example, research published in *Diabetes Care*[ix] presents the synergistic effects of GLP-1 receptor agonists and nutrition therapy resulting in improved glycemic control and reduced A1C levels for those with type-2 diabetes.

A seminal study published in *Endocrinology, Diabetes & Metabolism* in 2019[x] introduces the innovative concept of IDEP (Interaction between Diet/Exercise and Pharmacotherapy), suggesting that modifications in diet and lifestyle, along with medications, can yield favorable outcomes in patients with type-2 diabetes. This multi-prong approach can be used to promote the use of dietary interventions, exercise, and GLP-1 inhibitor therapy to manage diabetes, instead of just a singular intervention, such as medication.

Also, it must be noted that GLP-1 receptor agonists have side effects—most not so pleasant. Common side effects include nausea, vomiting, diarrhea, constipation, GERD, abdominal pain, dizziness, and hypoglycemia. Additionally, there can be concerns related to malnutrition and loss of muscle mass.

Don't worry; we are here to help you manage the side effects!

Let's be real, GLP-1 receptor agonists have been gaining increased attention and usage because they are effective in producing weight loss, as well as improved A1C levels.

The fusion of GLP-1 r receptor agonists and nutrition intervention can offer a pathway towards the prevention and management of chronic disease. So, embark on this journey with me, and step-by-step, you can discover improved health and a better quality of life. Let's get started!

Chapter 1 Summary:

- GLP-1 receptor agonists including exenatide (Byetta®, Bydureon®), liraglutide (Victoza®, Saxenda®), dulaglutide (Trulicity®), semaglutide (Ozempic®, Wegovy®), tirzepatide (Mounjaro®), and lixisenatide (Adlyxin®) have emerged as pharmacological treatments for type-2 diabetes and weight loss.

- These medications mimic the action of the naturally occurring hormone GLP-1, which regulates blood sugar levels and appetite.

- GLP-1 promotes insulin secretion, inhibits glucagon release, slows gastric emptying, and can have cardiovascular benefits.

- Tirzepatide and semaglutide are the most popularly prescribed GLP-1 receptor agonists, but they are different. The main difference is that tirzepatide mimics two hormones (GLP-1 and GIP) while semaglutide mimics one (GLP-1).

- Nutrition education plays a crucial role in optimizing health outcomes associated with GLP-1 receptor agonists by improving diet quality and overall health through diet and lifestyle modifications.

- Healthy eating habits, regular physical activity, and behavioral strategies, when combined with GLP-1 receptor agonists, can enhance long-term success in weight management and metabolic health.

- Nutrition education can help manage side affects associated with GLP-1 receptor agonists.

CHAPTER 2: THE POWER OF FIVE

MyPlate

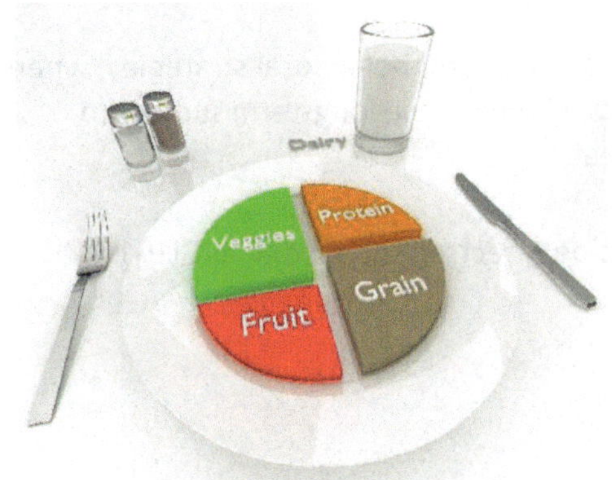

MyPlate is the United States Department of Agriculture's (USDA) program that acts as a guide as to what healthy eating patterns should look like. The premise is that if you change your diet to look like their plate illustration, you will be improving your health bite by bite.

This chapter is the foundation of nutrition education. No matter where you are in terms of your health, this chapter will help you understand how to balance your nutrition.

For people taking GLP-1 receptor agonists, there are specific reasons why this chapter applies to you. When your appetite decreases and your food intake reduces, it can be extremely difficult to eat whole, balanced meals and meet your daily nutrient requirements, such as fiber and protein. This chapter will teach you how to eat enough.

A recent study found that "Restraint eating may increase the sensitivity to the treatment effects of GLP-1,"[xi] and although reducing the amount you eat can be viewed as a benefit for those who are trying to lose weight, it is still essential to make sure you are getting the nutrients your body needs daily to prevent issues such as an altered metabolism or even malnutrition.

The Five Food Groups

I use the concept of the USDA MyPLate, but I call it something different. I call it the Power of Five. These five food groups are what your body needs to function; they power the cells in your body. With these five food groups, you can get all the vitamins, minerals, and nutrients your body needs to function optimally.

Adopting a balanced diet rich in fruits, vegetables, lean proteins, healthy fats, and whole grains supports weight-loss efforts.

My approach to MyPlate emphasizes the most nutrient-dense foods. I specify the importance of whole grains, and when it comes to dairy, I recommend low-fat dairy. I introduce plant-based proteins in the protein category but provide lean meat choices too. You do not have to be a vegetarian; you can even eat steak and follow this program. That said, this program will work for vegetarians too!

I developed the Power of Five concept when I was a single mom. At the time, my girls were five and seven. Mornings were crazy getting them ready for school. If you are a parent, I am sure you know how stressful mornings can be. I wanted their lunches to be nutritious, and I wanted them to know the importance of getting the Power of Five in their lunches, so I educated them and allowed them to pack their own lunches.

I would ask them each if they had all their "parts" in their lunch, and they always did. An example would be a whole grain turkey sandwich with avocado, a Greek yogurt, baby carrots, and grapes.

Recently, my youngest, now seventeen, was coming home fatigued every day. I asked her what she was eating for lunch, and she said most days she orders a turkey panini. I reminded her about her parts! She was missing veggies and healthy fats! My girl was not getting enough fiber! She started packing her own lunches again with all the parts and *voila*, she was feeling energized and more focused.

So why are all five food groups so important?

I'll share a fun story with you. Kelly's Choice is currently working with the New York State prison system. We made sure that there was a fruit, a vegetable, a protein, a grain, and a dairy product at each meal. Prior to us working with them, the inmates were mainly eating a lot of carbohydrates. By giving them the Power of Five, the inmates felt so much better. One of the main reasons for this is that their blood-sugar levels became balanced. As a matter of fact, a significant number of inmates who were coming in with type-2 diabetes, have since been able to discontinue their medication because their A1C levels became within normal range!

Food works synergistically. They need each other to power your body! For example, say you have a steak for dinner (an excellent iron provider. If you have strawberries on your plate (high in vitamin C, those little berries will help the steak's iron get absorbed into your bloodstream. Vitamin C helps your body absorb iron. Pretty cool, right?!

I don't want you to feel overwhelmed by all this. Before starting this program, most people don't get all five food groups in every meal. This program is a process!

Serving Sizes

If you haven't done so already, I want you to start looking at serving sizes on food labels. Don't look at fat, calories, carbs, or anything else right now. I want you to *only* look at serving sizes. You may be surprised!

Nutrition Facts	
Serving size 1 potato (148g/5.2oz)	
Amount per serving	
Calories	**110**
	% Daily Value*
Total Fat 0g	**0%**
Saturated Fat 0g	**0%**
Trans Fat 0g	
Cholesterol 0mg	**0%**
Sodium 0mg	**0%**
Total Carbohydrate 26g	**9%**
Dietary Fiber 2g	**7%**
Total Sugars 1g	
Includes 0g Added Sugars	**0%**
Protein 3g	
Vitamin D 0g	0%
Calcium 20mg	2%
Iron 1.1mg	6%
Potassium 620mg	15%
Vitamin C 27mg	30%
Vitamin B_6 0.2mg	10%

* The % Daily Value (DV) tells you how much a nutrient in a serving of food contributes to a daily diet. 2,000 calories a day is used for general nutrition advice.

At one of my workplace wellness events, we were all eating lunch together in an auditorium. A manager in the audience called me over and showed me his bag of cookies. He said, "I don't believe this! I have one of these bags of cookies every day, and each bag has three servings. This tiny little bag is three servings!"

This manager had not looked at the serving size on the label before this lesson, so he thought he was getting a certain number of grams of fat, calories, etc. from this package of cookies. But what he actually had to do was multiply the calories, the fat, the protein, and everything on the label by three!

So then, what about food without labels? There's a way you can determine food servings with something you have with you every day! Can you guess what it is?

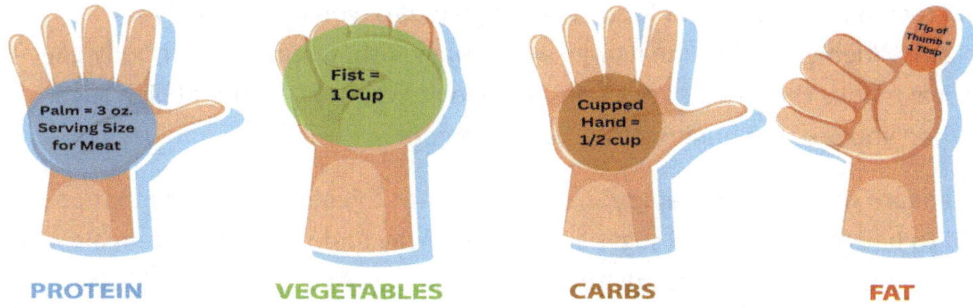

YOUR HAND. Here are some rules of "thumb" to use:

- A fist = 1 cup
- The palm of your hand = 3 oz.
- The tip of your thumb = 1 tbsp
- The tip of your pointer finger = 1 tsp
- A cupped hand = ½ cup

Here are some examples for you: -

- A serving of nuts should be ¼ cup so that's half of your cupped hand.
- A serving of meat should be 3-4 oz., so look at the palm of your hand for that.
- A good serving size for peanut butter is usually 1-2 tablespoons, so look to your thumb tip for that.
- And when you want to fry an egg, look at your pointer fingertip to see how much oil to add to your pan.

Eat Balanced Meals

So many people I have worked with skip meals. Maybe they're in a rush in the morning or not hungry, so they skip breakfast. Or, they have meetings all day, so they skip lunch. I do not want you to do this! I recommend that you have three balanced meals a day, trying your best to incorporate the Power of Five. There are a couple quick and easy recipes at the end of this chapter that can provide inspiration.

And get this: I am also recommending a snack each day.

Why am I recommending all this food? If you skip meals, you can disrupt your metabolism. When you skip a meal or go a long time without eating, your body goes into survival mode. This causes your cells and body to crave high fat and high sugar foods. When you are that hungry often, anything goes.

Have you heard of the word "hangry"? You don't want to get your body to that point. You need to balance your blood sugar and the best way to do this is to eat meals with all five food groups and to eat regularly throughout the day. An example would be breakfast at 7-9 AM, lunch between 12 and 1 PM, a snack between 3 and 4 PM and dinner between 6 and 7 PM. That is ideal; it doesn't need to be exact.

Picture your metabolism as a blazing fire, fueled by the wood you provide, which represents your food intake. Just like a fire's flame dwindles when the wood deteriorates, your metabolism can slow down and ultimately fade away. To sustain that energetic flame—your metabolism—it's crucial to feed it consistently throughout the day.

There is science behind the way that unbalanced meals slow down your metabolism and how a slower metabolism can cause weight gain and increased belly fat, both of which are risk factors for type-2 diabetes and heart disease.

In one study, researchers from Japan[xii] investigated close to 800 participants' eating patterns between 2011 and 2013. They found that those who skipped breakfast were the most likely to have an increased waist circumference and weight gain. Skipping breakfast can disrupt your appetite and blood sugar regulation, leading to cravings and overconsumption throughout the later parts of the day.

My patient Michael had type-2 diabetes and he went through this same program you are going through. He always skipped breakfast or simply had a cup of coffee. He started having a scrambled egg and a piece of whole grain toast for breakfast or sometimes peanut butter on whole grain toast. Within a month, he lost 8 pounds, and he expressed feeling so much better. He said, "I couldn't believe how much more energy I had and how much better I was able to concentrate by having breakfast."

Yep, it's true. Skipping breakfast negatively impacts your energy levels; the lack of food signals your body to shut things down (like brain function). Consuming a little bit of protein and whole grain recharges your cells and your body. You are supposed to break the fast for breakfast!

And remember that fire! It's important to avoid skipping any meal!

I was at the bank a few months ago, and my banker told me how she never has time to eat lunch, so she's ravenous when she gets home and snacks like crazy while she is making dinner. This habit has been detrimental to her weight-loss and health goals. I told her about the five parts and advised her to try it for lunch on just a couple "slower" days a week. I saw her the other day and she informed me that she gets all parts for lunch every day now. She looked radiant and had reached her desired weight!

A patient of mine, Kim, came to me with massive, crippling reflux symptoms. Kim works a 9-5 job during the day and cleans houses at night. In between her day job and her night job, she would have a candy bar to hold her over and then she would do some late-night snacking when she got home.

We had her switch her candy bar to a salad with some protein, and she gave herself twenty extra minutes to eat between her jobs. This satiated her, and she didn't crave snacks late at night. Within two weeks, her reflux was gone for good.

Chapter 2 Summary:

- MyPlate, a program by the USDA, can be used as a tool to visualize and balance food groups on your plate, which can improve health gradually over time.

- GLP-1 receptor agonists decrease your appetite, reducing your caloric intake, resulting in weight loss. When this weight loss is significant and rapid, you can be at an increased risk for malnutrition.

- The Power of Five emphasizes the consumption of foods from five essential food groups: fruits, vegetables, lean proteins, whole grains, and dairy products. This balanced and realistic approach promotes nutrient-dense foods, rather than focusing on restriction and exclusion in your diet.

- Understanding serving sizes, whether from food labels or using hand measurements, can help individuals make informed choices and avoid overconsumption.

- Balanced meals containing all five food groups throughout the day help maintain steady blood sugar and energy levels and prevent metabolic slowdown.

- Skipping meals, especially breakfast, can disrupt metabolism and lead to weight gain; incorporating balanced meals and snacks at regular intervals supports energy levels and overall health.

Chapter 2 Goals:

As a reminder, at the end of each chapter, you will have goals to accomplish before moving on to the next chapter. These goals build off each other—the goal areas are in nutrition, fitness, and hydration.

Nutrition Goal

You have three goals in this section.

1.) Your first nutrition goal is to start looking at your serving sizes—read your food labels and use the "hand" secret. Remember, you don't have to be perfect; you will be educated more as we go along.

2.) Your second goal is to start keeping a food journal. Try an app if it is easier! Being aware of what you're eating, and your eating patterns are the first steps to success.

3.) Try at least one of the recipes in this book.

Exercise Goals

Begin incorporating daily movement via stretching in the morning. Reach for your toes. Stretch your arms as high as you can.

Hydration

I haven't talked much about this, but hydration is a crucial part of your success. See Appendix A for some self-hydration tests you can try!

I had my patient Cindy try some of these self-tests when she complained of headaches. She was very dehydrated; she was pondering her water intake and joked that she can't remember any time in the past year that she drank a full glass of water.

Did you know that you should drink water even before you feel thirsty? Thirst is an emergency response from your body!

We are going to build up on hydration. For now just make sure you drink *some* water every day, if even just a glass!

Work on this chapter for as long as you feel comfortable, and when you are ready, you can move on to Chapter 2 where we will focus on carbohydrates.

Sheet Pan Chicken & Veggies

Serves 4 people

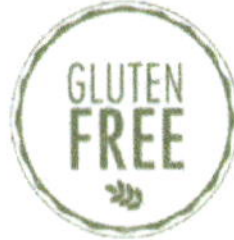

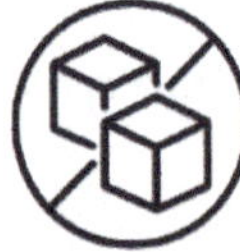
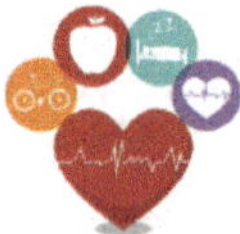
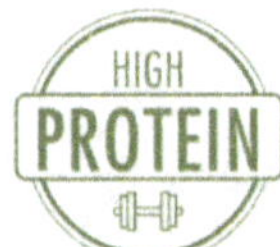

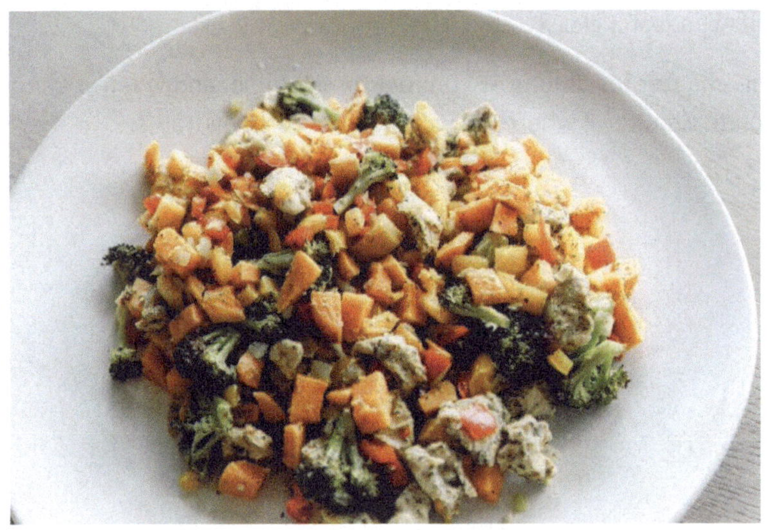

Ingredients:

- 1 lb. chicken breasts, diced
- 4 medium sized sweet potatoes, diced
- 1 large onion, diced
- 2 bell peppers, diced
- 2 cups broccoli florets, chopped
- 1/4 cup avocado oil
- 1/2 tsp. salt
- 1 tsp. pepper
- 1 tsp. garlic powder
- 1 tsp. dried thyme
- 1 tsp. dried oregano

Directions:

Preheat oven to 400 degrees F. While the oven preheats, add chicken, sweet potatoes, onion, bell pepper, and broccoli to a mixing bowl. Add avocado oil and seasonings. Stir until evening coated. Lightly coat a non-stick sheet pan with avocado oil. Pour the chicken and vegetable mixture onto pan and spread out evenly. Bake for 40-50 minutes, or until crispy. If you are looking for a heartier meal.Serve hot over whole grain, such as brown rice or quinoa.

Turkey Meatballs in Tomato Basil Sauce
Serves 4

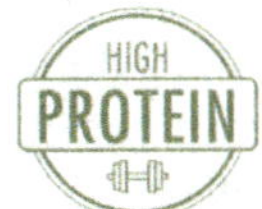

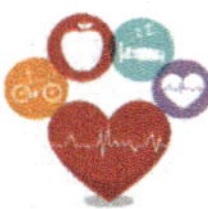
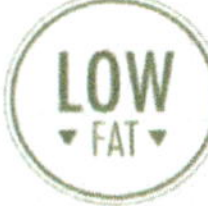

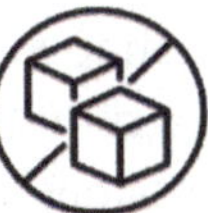

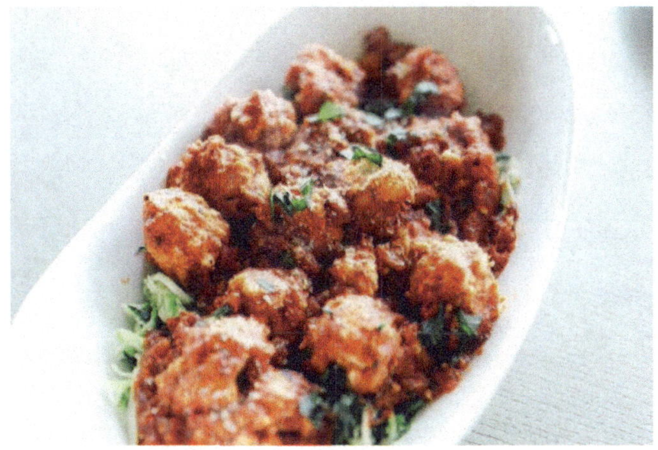

Ingredients for Tomato Basil Sauce

- 1 tbsp. olive oil
- 2 garlic cloves, finely chopped
- 1/4 tsp. crushed red pepper flakes
- 2 Tbsp. tomato paste
- 28 oz. crushed tomatoes, no salt added
- 1 large fresh basil sprig
- 1/4 tsp. salt

Ingredients for Turkey Meatballs

- 1/2 cup skim milk
- 1/2 cup panko breadcrumbs
- 1 large egg
- 1.5 oz. grated parmesan cheese
- 1/4 cup fresh parsley, chopped
- 1/2 tsp. dried oregano
- 1 tsp. salt
- 1 lb. lean ground turkey, 95%

Directions

Heat olive oil over medium heat in a large skillet. Add the garlic and red pepper flakes. Cook for about 1 minute. Add in tomato paste and keep stirring for about 2 minutes, until color turns orange. Pour in crushed tomatoes and salt. Bring to a simmer and add basil. Continue to simmer while preparing the meatballs.

Combine the breadcrumbs, milk, egg, cheese, parsley, oregano and salt to a large mixing bowl. Stir until well-blended. Add the ground turkey and use fork or hand to mix until well-combined. Wet hands and shape into 1-inch balls. Mixture should make about 22-24 meatballs. Place meatballs in tomato sauce, cover skillet, and cook for 20 minutes until meatballs are thoroughly cooked. Garnish with basil and enjoy!

CHAPTER 3: GETTING TO KNOW CARBOHYDRATES

Carbohydrates are the most prevalent nutrient in the diet because they come from so many different sources. Whenever you see the words sugar or fiber, these are carbohydrates! We're going to break down carbs in this lesson so that you understand which ones are best for your body and why.

Carbs are a hotly debated topic. Many patients have come to me thinking they should avoid or limit carbs like many diets such as Atkins, South Beach, and the Keto Diet suggest. As I mentioned in the introduction, I do not believe in deprivation, and the truth is that you *need* carbohydrates!

Carbohydrates are how you give your body energy and fuel. When talking about carbs, we are going to be focusing on the sources and amount of energy you are giving your body to optimize energy levels, nutrient intake, and blood sugar management.

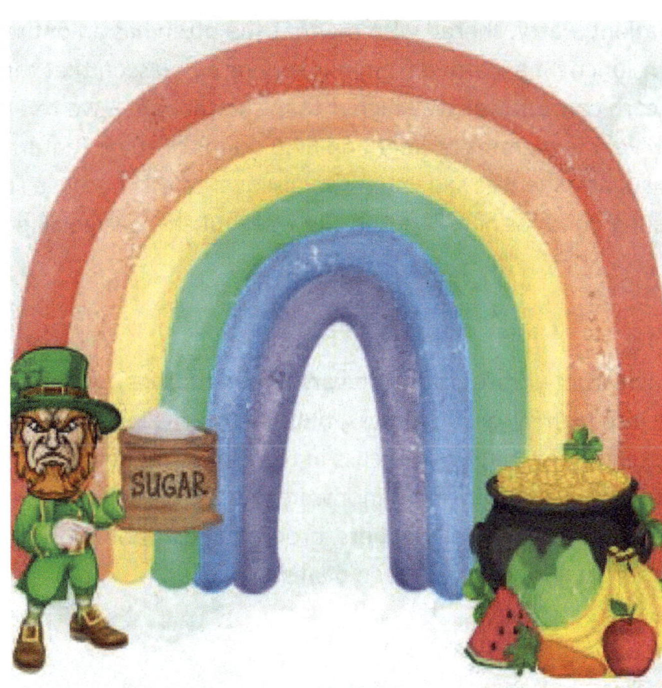

The Rainbow of Carbohydrates

I want you to think of carbohydrates as a spectrum, a giant rainbow. One side has a pot of gold, and the other side has a very angry leprechaun. Carbs are like a rainbow because so many different food sources contain carbs! The obvious sources would be bread, pasta, rice, and sweets. The less obvious sources are dairy, legumes, and starchy vegetables.

The pot of gold end has fiber-rich, complex carbs that come from veggies, fruits, legumes, and whole grains. The leprechaun end has processed foods: white bread, white pasta, white rice, cakes, cookies, crackers, ice-cream, jams...the list goes on!

The leprechaun is mischievous and wants you to have some of his food, which makes you crave it. Everything goes in moderation, but we want to go toward the pot of gold side more than the leprechaun side.

Let's dive into the pot of gold. The "gold" carbs are complex carbs, fiber-rich choices.

Fruit

Fruits are loaded with antioxidants; they are so good for you, and that is why they are on the "Power of Five" team. But we do have to keep in mind that fruits are carbs, and we should not go overboard because they do have sugar. Yes, it's natural sugar, But again, everything in moderation.

I'll give you an example. My patient, Patty, shared with me that she often has an entire can of pineapples every day for lunch. She learned from our serving size lesson that the can had 4.5 servings, and the carb content was way higher than she thought—we're talking 81 grams of carbs, with very few grams of fiber and 67.5 grams of sugar (natural sugar, not added, but still, it's sugar). She was sad when she discovered this because she thought she was doing something *good* for her diet. And she was, but she was getting too much!

Vegetables

Most vegetables are very low in carbohydrates, but some are high. Potatoes, winter squash, and peas, for instance, are high in carbohydrates, but despite this fact, there are some amazing nutrients in these veggies that I will discuss in the Fruits and Veggies chapter. I recommend trying to get all colors of the rainbow in your veggie selection. Some of my favorite low-carb vegetables are bell peppers, broccoli, mushrooms, zucchini, asparagus, leafy greens, cauliflower, and green beans.

Whole Grains

Whole grains, also carbohydrates, are a great way to get your fiber. There is a vast variety of whole grains, but here are some that I often recommend:

- Whole-grain wheat
- Oats
- Farro
- Millet
- Quinoa
- Buckwheat
- Barley
- Wild rice
- Amaranth

A lot of these whole grains come pre-packaged with instructions. When you shop your whole grain aisle, you want to look for whole grains that don't have a long list of ingredients. If you haven't heard of some of these grains, even better! Incorporating new foods is a great way to add a variety of nutrients to your diet and get creative in the kitchen! No one wants to eat the same thing for dinner every night! Switch it up by using different whole grains.

At the end of this chapter and at the end of the book, you will find some fun and easy recipes using these grains.

What about Bread?

Now, bread can be tricky. You want to make sure it's whole grain, but the marketing can easily fool you. So, let's look at what makes a grain whole.

Anatomy of a grain

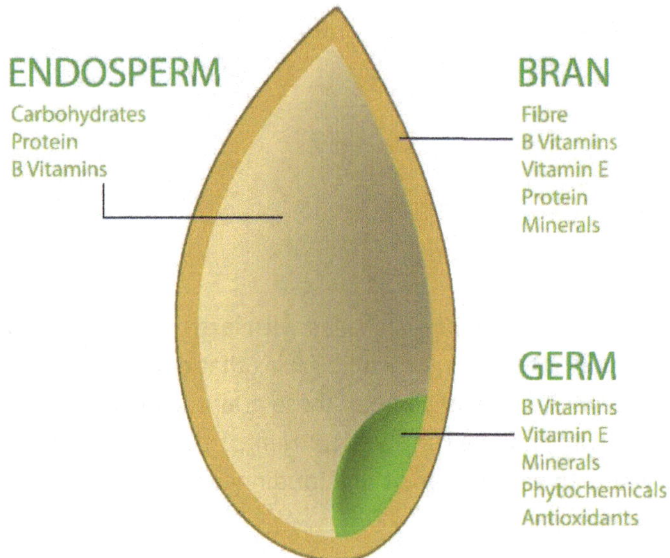

A whole grain has three parts: the bran, the germ, and the endosperm. The bran and germ are packed with fiber and B vitamins. You're left with the endosperm that is mostly made up of starch (which breaks down like a simple sugar). Refined foods like white bread or oyster crackers have no fiber because they are processed by stripping out the bran and germ.

At Kelly's Choice, we have kids (and adults too) conduct an experiment using orange juice to discover the difference between whole grains and refined grains. You're probably thinking, "What the heck? You use orange juice?" But hear me out.

We have them pour orange juice over a piece of white bread and then pour it over a piece of whole grain bread. The white bread dissolves into mush within seconds, and it takes quite some time for the whole grain bread to dissolve. This is what is happening in your stomach! The orange juice mimics stomach acid. Refined grains like white bread dissolve quickly, making you hungry faster. The whole grain dissolves much slower because the fiber is holding it together.

So, when you are buying bread, make sure it says 100% whole wheat or 100% whole grain. At the very least, make sure whole wheat or whole grain are the very first ingredients.

Be mindful. I am a smart bread shopper, but even I was tricked before. My girls were having hot dogs at a family barbeque. I went out to buy better hot dog buns. They looked hearty and were light brown, so I assumed they were whole wheat! But upon reading the label later in the day, I learned that they were NOT whole wheat and contained about eighteen processed ingredients.

How many carbs should I have?

One of the main things to consider in this transformation journey is how to stabilize blood sugar levels. if you keep your blood sugar stable throughout the day, I promise you aren't going to have as many cravings; you are going to be satisfied and successful!

While your GLP-1 receptor agonist medication can help manage blood-sugar levels, fiber will give you additional support. If you get to the point where you no longer need your medication, fiber along with your balanced plate should be your go-tos for managing blood-sugar levels.

Science supports the importance of fiber in GLP-1 secretion.

In a 2016 study, scientists determined that foods rich in nutrients such as high-fiber grain products, "seem to influence GLP-1 secretion and may thus promote associated beneficial outcomes in healthy individuals as well as individuals with type 2 diabetes or with other metabolic disturbances"[xiii]

We want to make sure we are getting carbohydrates *with fiber* consistently throughout the day. Start looking at food labels and gauging how many carbohydrates you are getting in each meal. You don't have to do this forever, just do this for this week so you can start familiarizing yourself with carbohydrates.

I want to see if you can get 30-45 grams of carbs at breakfast,30- 45 grams at lunch, and 30-45 grams at dinner. Many online apps can help you calculate these! It doesn't need to be exact—aim to get close to this range each meal. If you are taking GLP-1 medication, consuming this amount may be difficult, and that's okay.

Consuming carbs with fiber for your meals and snacks can help to stabilize your blood sugar levels and provide your body with sustainable energy throughout the day.

Paying Attention to Fiber

Now that you know the grams of carbohydrates to aim for in each meal, let's add fiber to the equation. You should try to get *at least* 7-10 grams of fiber per meal. The typical American only gets 10-15 grams of fiber a day. USDA's recommended daily amount of fiber for adults up to age 50 is between 25 grams for women and 38 grams for men. For adults older than 50, the recommendation is between 21 and 30 grams. Remember that the pot of gold foods provide this much-needed fiber.

There are two types of fiber: soluble and insoluble. When soluble fiber dissolves, it creates a gel that helps improve digestion. These fibers absorb water, increase stool bulk, and lower blood sugar and cholesterol levels. Insoluble fiber helps soften the stool because it attracts water into your stool; this prevents constipation and keeps your intestines healthy.

Excellent sources of soluble fiber include fruits like apples, grapefruits, and oranges, as well as beans, lentils, peas, oats, oat bran, and barley.

And excellent types of insoluble fiber include vegetables and whole grains like wheat, quinoa, stone ground cornmeal, bran, buckwheat, and brown rice.

Think of fiber like a kitchen sponge. You have the green scratch pad on one side and the yellow sponge on the other side. Insoluble fiber is the green scratchy side because it scrubs and cleans things up. Soluble fiber is the sponge side, mopping everything up.

Research shows that both types of fiber can decrease your risk of death from both cancer and heart disease.

In one study, for example,[xiv] the dietary habits and health of more than 160,000 women were followed for up to 18 years. The women who consumed an average of 2-3 servings of whole grains a day were 30% less likely to have developed type-2 diabetes than those who rarely ate whole grains.

One of the most groundbreaking studies was published in the *Lancet* peer-reviewed journal in 2019.[xv] This study was a review using data from 185 prospective studies and 58 clinical trials. The researchers found that eating fiber from a variety of whole foods can decrease the risk of death from heart disease, stroke, type-2 diabetes, and/or colon cancer by up to 24%, compared to people who eat very little fiber.

If you wean off from GLP-1 medications, fiber is my number-one recommendation for you. Frank Duca, who studies metabolic diseases at the University of Arizona, claims that foods with fiber are the best food choices for increasing the production of GLP-1 naturally.[xvi] Fiber will help you keep up the production of GLP-1.

In addition to increasing the production of GLP-1s naturally, fiber also helps to lower your cholesterol and blood pressure—it protects your heart![xvii]

Fiber helps with weight loss because you will feel full longer. When you first start eating enough fiber, you may feel bloated, but don't let that fool you! That will eventually go away; your body is just getting used to eating fiber. Also, you should increase water intake as you increase fiber to avoid constipation. A five-minute walk after your meal will help your digestion as well.

How can you get over 25 grams of fiber into your day?

Let's look at a typical day to see how to do this.

At breakfast, options could include one of the following: a slice of whole grain toast, oatmeal, granola (but make sure the added sugar is less than 10 grams and that the fiber is at least 4 grams), or some fruit. At lunch, fiber may be in your whole grain sandwich bread or the vegetables in your salad or a piece of fruit. At dinner, your veggies and a whole grain like quinoa or farro will give you a lot of fiber.

My patient Michael started replacing French fries at dinner with broccoli. French fries are often a carb overload and have little to no fiber while broccoli has 6.6 grams of carbohydrates with 2.8 grams of that being fiber! Michael then added a half of cup of a whole grain rice with his dinner, and he easily reaches his goal of carbs and fiber!

Nutrition Facts	
Serving size 1 potato (148g/5.2oz)	
Amount per serving	
Calories	**110**
	% Daily Value*
Total Fat 0g	0%
Saturated Fat 0g	0%
Trans Fat 0g	
Cholesterol 0mg	0%
Sodium 0mg	0%
Total Carbohydrate 26g	9%
Dietary Fiber 2g	7%
Total Sugars 1g	
Includes 0g Added Sugars	0%
Protein 3g	
Vitamin D 0g	0%
Calcium 20mg	2%
Iron 1.1mg	6%
Potassium 620mg	15%
Vitamin C 27mg	30%
Vitamin B_6 0.2mg	10%

* The % Daily Value (DV) tells you how much a nutrient in a serving of food contributes to a daily diet. 2,000 calories a day is used for general nutrition advice.

So, here's how you look for carbohydrates and fiber on an ingredient label In bold, you will see the total number of carbohydrates. Then below it, you will have fiber, sugar, and added sugar. You want to look for foods with fiber. Four grams of fiber is an ideal goal in most food choices. You want to look for little to no added sugar *most of the time.* Remember, you're developing healthy habits here. You don't have to restrict yourself from anything; just make sure that you choose wisely most of the time.

My patient Kenny said, "I don't deny myself things. My poor choices are calculated and limited. I try to balance it out through the course of the day. I try to eliminate things that don't have fiber. It's almost a hobby now."

Remember, we're working to stabilize blood sugar. Here's a food example: Chinese food! Do you ever crave it? I do, but I have learned to replicate it at home. I like chicken dishes. Most Chinese places only offer you a choice of fried rice or white rice. Many of my patients think they are making a healthy choice by selecting the white rice, but the fact is that white rice will spike your blood sugar. About the only time I recommend white rice is when recovering from a cold or flu.

So, this is how I create my rendition of a Chinese meal. I swap the white rice with brown rice. That is step one in avoiding a blood sugar spike. And then the added chicken (a protein source) and broccoli (a fiber source) with various spices instead of a sugary sauce does a beautiful job at satiating me and satisfies my Chinese food craving! You can explore other options too—try wild rice, quinoa, or black rice—all are excellent as the carbohydrate portion of your stir-fry!

A plethora of research suggests that my experiment will help protect me from type-2 diabetes and other chronic conditions. For example, a 2013 study published in the *European Journal of Epidemiology*[xviii] concluded that replacing refined grains with whole grains and eating at least two servings of whole grains daily may help to reduce type-2 diabetes risk. The reason why is because the fiber and nutrients in whole grains may slow the absorption of food, helping to prevent blood sugar spikes.

Food marketing can be tricky! The angry leprechaun also owns some not-so-obvious unhealthy food choices. For example, my patient Allie was obsessed with almond crackers; she figured they were a healthy choice and assumed they were high in fiber. After all, almonds were in her handy high-fiber food chart. But a serving of these processed crackers only had 1 gram of fiber of the 24 grams of carbohydrates in a serving. Allie always felt tired and hungry; it's no wonder—her snack of choice was spiking her blood sugar, and then it would plummet.

Now, turning to the pot of gold side: when you choose those foods like whole grains, beans, and most veggies, your blood sugar will remain stable.

Check out the chart that Allie and all my patients use for some great fiber choices (when they are in their natural form) and if you need some inspiration for using these choices, the included recipes will definitely help!

High-Fiber Foods Checklist:

- **Raw Nuts & Seeds**
    - Chia Seeds: 19.5 grams per cup (great in yogurt, oatmeal, or smoothies!)
    - Ground Flaxseed: 11.5 grams per ¼ cup (also great in yogurt, oatmeal, or smoothies!)
    - Almonds: 4.5 grams per ¼ cup
    - Pistachios: 3.25 grams per ¼ cup
    - Sunflower Seeds: 3 grams per ¼ cup
    - Walnuts: 2 grams per ¼ cup
- **Cooked Whole Grains**
    - Hulled Barley: 31.8 grams per cup
    - Teff: 7 grams per cup
    - Brown Rice: 6.7 grams per cup
    - Quinoa: 5.2 grams per cup
    - Buckwheat: 4.5 per cup
    - Farro: 3 grams per cup
- **Cooked Leafy Greens**
    - Collard Greens: 5.6 grams per cup
    - Kale: 4.7 grams per cup
    - Spinach: 4 .7 grams per cup

- Swiss Chard: 3.7 grams per cup
- Cabbage: 2.8 grams per cup

- **Raw Leafy Greens**
  - Cabbage: 4.4 grams per cup
  - Collard Greens: 2.9 grams per cup
  - Kale: 1.7 grams per cup
  - Swiss Chard: 1.2 grams per cup
  - Spinach: 1.1 grams per cup
- **More Veggies**
  - Baked Acorn Squash: 9 grams per cup
  - Cooked Peas: 8.3 grams per ½ cup
  - Cooked Brussels Sprouts: 4 grams per cup
  - Cooked Broccoli: 3.2 grams per cup
  - Cooked Cauliflower: 2.9 grams per cup
- **Beans & Legumes**
  - Navy Beans: 19 grams per cup
  - Adzuki Beans: 16.8 grams per cup
  - Lentils: 15.6 grams per cup
  - Black Beans: 15 grams per cup
  - Lima Beans: 13.2 grams per cup
  - Chickpeas: 12.5 grams per cup
  - Kidney Beans: 11.3 grams per cup
- **Fruit**
  - Raspberries: 8 grams per cup
  - Blackberries: 7.6 grams per cup
  - Pears (1 medium size): 5.5 grams
  - Apple (1 medium): 4 grams
  - Blueberries: 3.6 grams per cup
  - Orange (1 medium): 3.4 grams

You may be wondering why the cooked leafy greens have more fiber than raw leafy greens. Think about it this way: To make a salad with raw spinach, you pull out enough spinach leaves from the container to equal two cups. Your bowl of salad has two cups of spinach leaves, but there is a lot of air between the leaves. To yield one cup of cooked spinach, you need to pull out many more cups of raw leaves, because when you cook leafy greens, they shrink. Despite the shrinkage, the fiber is still there!

Chapter 3 Summary:

- Carbohydrates are essential for providing energy to the body, but making wise choices is crucial for optimal health.

- Remember the rainbow analogy! The "pot of gold" side of the carbohydrate spectrum includes fiber-rich foods found in vegetables, fruits, and whole grains, which offer numerous health benefits. On the other hand, processed foods like white flour products, cakes, cookies, and ice cream represent the "angry leprechaun" side of the spectrum, offering little nutritional value and often leading to cravings and overconsumption.

- Fruits, while nutritious, should be consumed in moderation due to their natural sugar content, highlighting the importance of portion control. Aim for 2-3 servings a day.

- Vegetables, particularly those with vibrant colors, are low in carbohydrates and rich in essential nutrients, making them a cornerstone of a healthy diet.

- Whole grains, such as quinoa, farro, and oats, provide ample fiber and nutrients, offering a healthier alternative to refined grains.

- Understanding food labels is essential for making informed choices, with a focus on selecting products with higher fiber content and minimal added sugars.

- Fiber naturally increases GLP-1 production and lowers cholesterol and blood pressure.

- Incorporating fiber into each meal helps stabilize blood sugar levels and promotes satiety, contributing to overall health and weight management. It also supports a healthy gut and can aid in sustaining weight loss after weaning off these medications.

Chapter 3 Goals:

For this chapter, continue the goals from the last chapter and build off of them as we progress through this book.

Nutrition: For nutrition, continue paying attention to serving sizes. And now we're going to look at total grams of carbs and fiber. Remember you want to aim for 45 grams of carbohydrates per meal and 7-10 grams of fiber. Don't get stressed out about this counting—just familiarize yourself with getting the recommended amount of carbs and fiber in your meals. As I said in the introduction, this program is NOT about counting things; it's about educating you on how to create healthy habits. This initial counting is to create an awareness of proper portions —that's all.

And one other nutrition goal is to try a recipe from this chapter!

Fitness: Walk and stretch five minutes daily.

Hydration: Drink an 8-ounce glass of water right when you first wake up.

Broccoli Quinoa Salad
Serves 3-4 people

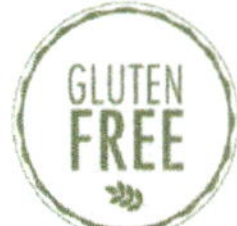

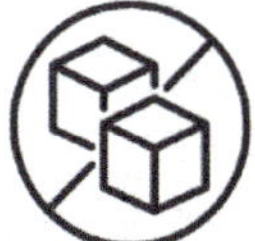
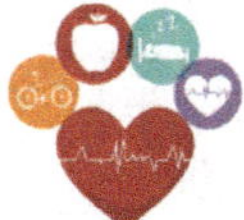
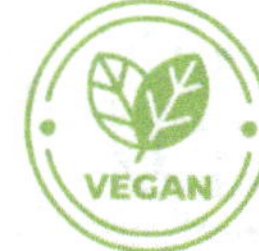

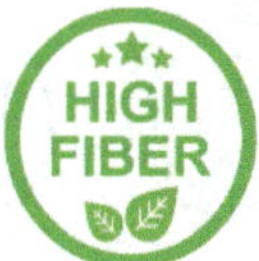

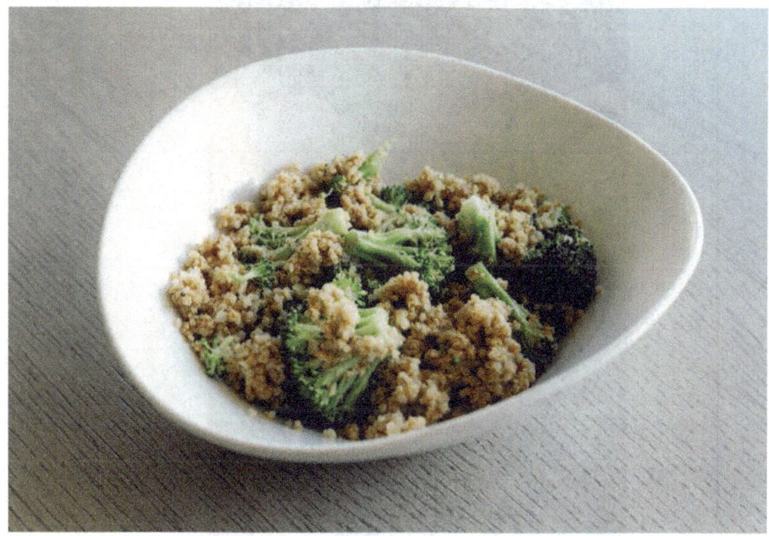

Ingredients

- 1/2 cup dry quinoa
- 2 heads of broccoli, finely chopped
- Juice from 4 lemons
- 2 Tbsp. avocado oil
- 1/2 cup tahini
- 1/2 tsp. Dijon mustard
- 1 tsp. garlic powder
- 1 tsp. onion powder
- 1 Tbsp. paprika
- 1/2 tsp. black pepper

Directions

Cook quinoa according to package. While the quinoa is cooking, remove the stems from the broccoli and finely chop. Add lemon juice, avocado oil, tahini, Dijon mustard, garlic powder, onion powder, paprika, and black pepper to a bowl. Wisk until smooth. Add additional water as necessary. In large bowl, combine cooked quinoa, broccoli and dressing. Toss thoroughly to coat. Serve warm or cold.

Easy Overnight Oats
Recipe makes one serving

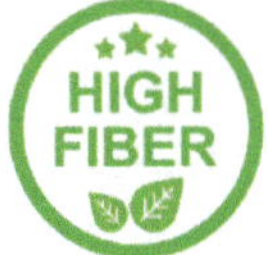

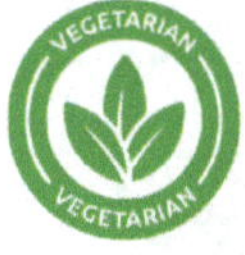

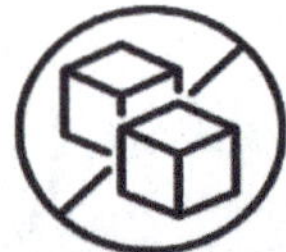
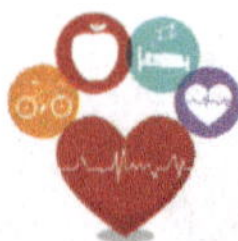
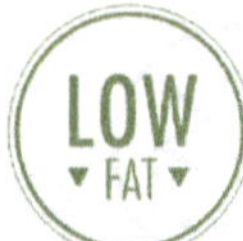

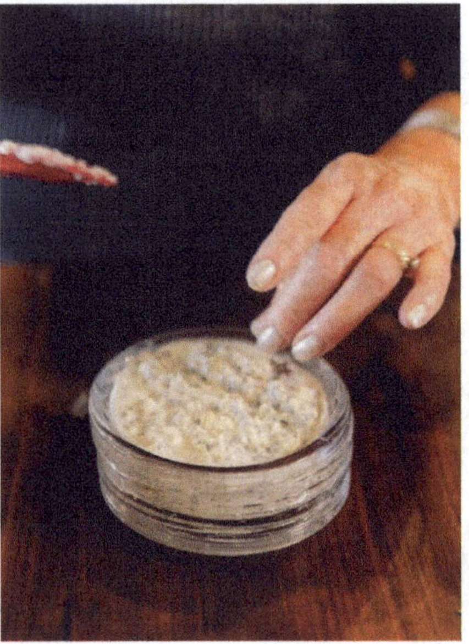

Ingredients

- 1/2 cup old-fashioned rolled oats
- 1/2 cup milk of choice
- 1/4 cup plain yogurt
- 2 tsp. honey or preferred sweetener of choice
- 2 tsp. chia seeds
- Pinch of salt
- Toppings of choice

Directions

Place oats, milk, yogurt, honey, chia seeds and salt in a jar or container. Mix the ingredients together with a spoon and seal the jar or container. Place the jar in the refrigerator and refrigerate overnight. The next day, remove the lid and stir the oats. If the consistency of the oats is too thick for your liking, add a little bit more milk to thin it out. Add toppings of your choosing to the oats and enjoy!

CHAPTER 4: POWERFUL PROTEIN

Chances are you have learned a little bit about protein from all the protein-focused diets like keto, Atkins®, or South Beach® . Don't worry, I am not going to have you start drinking protein shakes or follow *any* diet. As I have said before and will say again, this program is about education.

Protein carries nutrients to your cells! Protein also provides structure for your organs and tissues—everything from your bones and muscles to your skin and intestinal lining. Imagine your bloodstream as a canal—proteins are the cargo ships that carry vitamins, minerals, sugars, cholesterol, etc. where they are needed. These protein cargo ships sometimes "hold onto" nutrients like iron so you have a backup supply when you need it.

So, let's dive in and learn specifics about protein—there's a lot to learn!

Animal Protein vs. Plant Protein

I will start by talking about the two categories of protein—there is protein that comes from **animals** and proteins that come from **plants**.

Both types of protein are beneficial.

Animal protein is beneficial because it is more bioavailable (meaning it readily absorbed and used by the body) and has iron and B vitamins. It has no carbohydrates.

Plant proteins are important because they also have fiber (a word that you will hear again and again throughout this book), are lower in saturated fat, and have a plethora of vitamins and minerals.

I would love to see you have both on your plate (unless you are a vegetarian or vegan of course).

How Much Protein Do You Need?

In the Power of Five chapter, you learned that protein takes up about 25% of the plate. With protein, it is critical to remember that more is not better. Protein intake beyond your needs will likely store as fat. That is why it is so important to get it evenly throughout the day in the right amount. I recommend getting somewhere between 20 to 30 grams of protein per meal and around 5-10 grams for your snacks.

If you are taking GLP-1 receptor agonists, I suggest aiming for the higher end of my recommended grams of protein per meal. Increasing your protein intake can be crucial if you are trying to reduce your body fat percentage while preserving your lean muscle mass.

A 2021 published study by a team of professors in Japan[xix] found that those taking GLP-1 medication had experienced a decrease in the fat-free mass compared to others in the study who were taking a placebo. This means that some weight loss was not due to a reduction in body fat, but fat-free mass such as lean muscle tissues. Losing muscle mass is concerning, especially throughout the aging process. You need those muscles! You can help reduce or prevent the loss of fat-free mass by eating adequate protein through protein-focused meals and a variety of lean animal and plant-based protein sources.

Common Food Sources and Amount of Protein

Plant Protein Sources	**Grams of protein**
2 tablespoons Chia Seeds	4.7
2 tablespoons Flaxseeds	2.6
¼ cup Pumpkin Seeds	9.8
¼ cup Almonds	7.6
¼ cup Walnuts	3.8
¼ cup Cashews	10.3
¾ cup Quinoa	6
1 slice Whole Wheat Bread	4
½ cup Kidney Beans	6.7
½ cup Black Beans	7.3
½ cup Chickpeas	8.9
½ cup Green Peas	3.8
½ cup Lentils	9
½ cup Edamame	9.2
½ cup Pinto Beans	7.2
2 Tablespoons Peanut butter	7.7
Animal Protein Sources	
3 oz. Skinless Chicken Breast	25.2
3 oz. Skinless Turkey Breast	24

3 oz. 95% Lean Ground Beef	18.2
3 oz. Sirloin Steak	24
3 oz. Beef tenderloin	23.8
3 oz. Salmon	22.5
3 oz. Tuna	16
3 oz. Haddock	17
3 oz. Pork Tenderloin	25.8
3 oz. Elk	25.7
3 oz. Venison	25.7
3 oz. Bison	24.1
¾ cup Plain Low-Fat Greek yogurt	18.3
1 cup Skim Milk	8 .4
1 cup Low-Fat Kefir	9.2
1 oz. Low-Fat Cheddar Cheese	6.9
2 Large Eggs	14

Let's look at some ways to incorporate protein in your meals. Say for breakfast, you have two eggs and one slice of whole wheat toast; the eggs have 14 grams of protein and the toast has 4 grams of protein, so that will bring you to a total of 18 grams of protein. Now, let's look at a lunch with the ideal amount of protein. Think about a turkey sandwich: 3 ounces of turkey is 24 grams of protein, and the wheat bread will give you another 8 grams of protein; so again, you will have around 32 grams of protein. For dinner, you could have 3 ounces of salmon and green beans with a serving of quinoa; the two main sources of protein in this meal are salmon with 22.5 grams of protein and quinoa with 6 grams of protein. Total protein for that meal will be 23 grams of protein.

I know it may seem like I'm breaking my promise of you not having to count numbers; you may be overwhelmed with fiber, carbs, now protein!

Here's the thing though; this is an initial step to familiarize you with how much you need and where to get good sources! You won't have to count forever!

I've had several patients who have been overwhelmed with the initial "counting." Take Kristin for example; she came to me after being diagnosed with high cholesterol, and she also wanted to lose some weight, which would naturally happen with addressing her high cholesterol and upgrading her food choices .

After her third session with me, Kristin said, "I don't know if I can do this. I'm overwhelmed, always keeping a notebook nearby, and writing down this food has this this many grams of fiber...this many grams of carbohydrates...this many grams of protein. It's just too much."

I responded, "We don't have to take this approach. How about we just have some protein, some carbs, and some fiber at every meal?"

What I told Kristin—and I will tell you—is to go back to the plate image. Just keep your eye on the plate and acknowledge the Power of Five. And please realize that you absolutely do not need a gram scale! If counting stresses you out, don't do it. This program can still work for you!

Kristin was so relieved. So, if you are feeling the way Kristin did, you can try the approach I recommended for her and see if that seems more feasible for you.

Good Sources or Animal Protein

If you look at the protein sources in the chart I have provided, these are some protein sources I recommend. One drawback of a lot of animal protein is that it is high in saturated fat. In the next chapter, you will get a lot more education on fats and why saturated fat harms your health (and your waistline).

The sources of animal protein I recommend are a variety of lean sources. If you are at the grocery store and you are looking at ground beef, you will see different proportions and they are usually 80/20, 90/10, and 95/5, and now you may even be able to find 99/1 products. The first number is the percentage of protein and the second number is the percentage of fat. So, you want to choose the 95/5 ground beef, which is only 5% fat. Sometimes instead of saying 80/20, 90/10, or 95/5, the term "lean" will be used. For example, 95% lean.

As a registered dietitian, I am invited to places all over the world to learn about food. A few years ago, I had an opportunity to go to a beef farm in Kansas. I learned about the different types of leanness and fattiness of the cow. One fascinating thing that I learned is that the tenderloin, which is in the middle of the cow—it's this little, small part—is

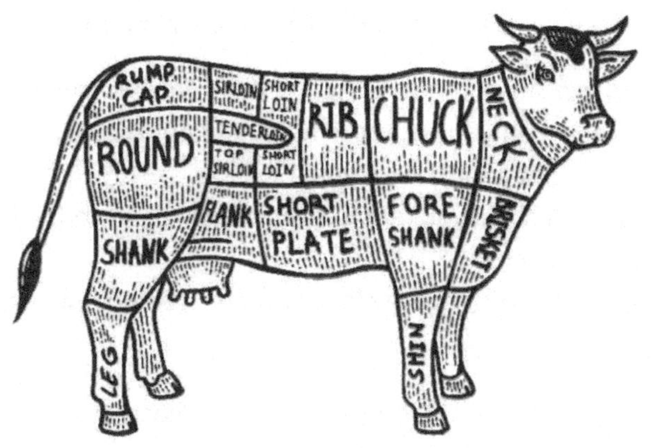

almost as lean as chicken. It's super, super lean! And then there are very fatty cuts of beef like brisket and prime rib.

When it comes to dairy products, I always recommend 2% or less for milk. For cheese, I recommend low-fat. Or part-skim.

One of the most common food indulgences that patients come to me with is cheese! They just don't want to give it up. I get it, low-fat cheese just doesn't taste the same! Here's my little secret…treat cheese as a condiment. Add just a sprinkling of a very flavorful cheese like Parmesan, Romano or extra-sharp cheese to salad, soups, and meat dishes too. It will fulfil your craving, I promise!

I have a meat recommendation that you may have not experienced—and that is game meat! I had one patient, James, who looked at me utterly confused when I mentioned game meat. He said, "So there are animals that are good at games?" I joked with him that deer are great at board games; he caught on and continued by saying he heard they were good at Scrabble.

In all seriousness, venison, bison, and elk are some of the leanest meats you can eat…hence why they are on my handy-dandy protein chart. They are free range, eating grasses and berries, and this in part is why they are so lean—not to mention, absolutely delicious! They are very high in iron, vitamin E, and selenium.

What's a Good Portion Size for Animal Protein?

What I have found is that most Americans are good at eating protein at dinner, but not at breakfast, lunch, or snack time. And while most people's protein consumption happens at dinner, the average American eats way too much protein.

A 2015 study[xx] found that the average American man consumes 100 grams of protein a day, and not evenly throughout the day. Do not save all your protein for dinner!

Eating protein regularly throughout the day is important for a few reasons:

- First, it helps your muscles grow and repair themselves, which is super important if you're active. When you eat protein throughout the day, your body always has what it needs to keep muscles strong.
- Having protein at every meal helps you feel full and satisfied, so you're less likely to overeat and gain weight.
- Having protein regularly keeps your energy levels steady, so you feel good all day long.

Look at the chart with recommended protein sources. As you will see, a 3 oz. sirloin steak has 24 grams of protein; most of us have been accustomed to eating at least double that—and six ounces of steak is 48 grams of protein- but not for some individuals who need even more protein per meal! Remember, what protein your body does not use at that mealtime will store as fat. This is why it is critical to spread out your protein sources evenly throughout your day.

Lean Meat Cooking Tip—You may not want to cook lean meats on the grill because they can dry out. I find that broiling lean meats is the perfect method—keeping them juicy and flavorful.

Good Sources of Plant Protein

Almonds and cashews and lentils and chickpeas; black beans and green peas, and flaxseeds, and quinoa; these are a few of my favorite things—when we are talking plant protein.

So, let's talk blood sugar and how plant proteins can help you balance blood sugar. The perfect example is apples with peanut butter. If you combine a plant protein with a carbohydrate, it will slow the release of sugar into your bloodstream. Neat, right?

What's a Good Portion Size for Plant Protein?

Generally, a quarter cup of nuts or seeds, a half cup of beans and legumes, and ¾ cup grains are good serving sizes for plant protein.

To get enough protein in a meal and keep it plant-based, you may need two sources, like beans and quinoa.

Digging a Little Bit Deeper—Amino Acids

Amino acids are the building blocks of protein. While there are 20 amino acids, nine of them are essential for your body to function optimally.

All animal proteins have every single one of those amino acids and very few plant proteins have all nine. Quinoa, buckwheat, soy, and amaranth are a few exceptions.

Any food that has all nine essential amino acids is called a complete protein.

However, if you do pairings with plant proteins, you can get all essential amino acids. The most popular example is brown rice and beans. These two buddies create a complete protein; together they have all nine essential amino acids. Here are some other plant protein pairings that create a complete protein:

- Whole wheat toast with peanut butter

- Hummus with whole grain tortilla chips

- Bean chili with bulgur wheat

- Chickpeas and sunflower seeds together in a spinach salad

- Almonds and oatmeal

- Peas and barley

While these are complete proteins, it does not mean you are getting all the nutrients you need. If you are vegan, it is very easy to become deficient in calcium, iron, vitamin D, vitamin K2, vitamin B12, and iodine. I recommend having your doctor order a blood test for all those levels, because deficiencies in those nutrients can lead to chronic conditions like osteoporosis.

It is possible to be a vegan, it just requires a lot of work and more education to make sure you are getting all the nutrients you need. See the Appendix B for vitamins and nutrients that vegans need to be mindful of.

Some of my patients have asked about taking amino acid supplements. Lysine is a popular one. That is not a good idea. Think of a pool of water that has nine water slides stemming from it. Each slide is designated to a particular amino acid. The pool is the holding area. If the pool becomes overfilled with an amino acid, like lysine...all the other water slides will shut down until much of the lysine goes down its slide...So sadly, your plan to repair your muscles with lysine backfires. These are called "essential" amino acids for a reason—you need all of them!

What Exactly Do the Nine Essential Amino Acids Do?

Amino Acid	Function
Histidine	Helps with brain function and produces red and white blood cells, important for overall health and immunity.
Isoleucine	Creates hemoglobin (which carries iron in the blood and helps regulate blood sugar, which is burned for energy in the muscles during exercise).
Leucine	Helps to stimulate muscle strength and retain lean muscle.
Lysine	Responsible for muscle repair and growth and may also help support immune system.
Methionine	Important for the growth of new blood vessels and muscles; it also contains Sulphur, which is integral to tissue health. Arthritis is a common result for people who do not consume enough Sulphur.
Phenylalanine	This amino acid actually turns into the amino acid tyrosine, which helps balance brain chemicals and therefore is tied to mood.
Threonine	Supports health function of immune system, liver, heart, and central nervous system.
Tryptophan	Tryptophan turns into serotonin, a neurotransmitter that can boost mood, lower depression and stress levels. It can also promote melatonin, which aids in sleep.
Valine	Responsible for muscle growth and repair; it also helps the central nervous system and cognitive function.

Chapter 4 Summary:

- Protein serves as a crucial nutrient for cellular function and structural support in the body, aiding in the transport of essential vitamins, minerals, and other nutrients.

- Animal protein, rich in iron and B vitamins, and plant protein, abundant in fiber and low in saturated fat, offer unique health benefits when included in the diet.

- The recommended protein intake per meal ranges from 20 to 30 grams, with protein consumption toward the higher end of this recommendation advised for individuals taking GLP-1 agonist receptor medications to support weight loss and muscle preservation.

- Plant protein sources, including nuts, seeds, legumes, and grains, offer diverse options for incorporating protein into meals while promoting blood sugar balance and satiety.

- Lean cuts of animal protein, such as skinless poultry, fish, lean beef and game meats like venison and elk, provide ample protein without excessive saturated fat intake, contributing to overall heart health.

- It's essential to distribute protein intake evenly throughout the day to optimize utilization and prevent excess protein storage as fat, aiming for appropriate portion sizes to meet daily nutritional needs.

- Plant protein combinations, such as beans and rice or hummus with whole grain chips, can provide all nine essential amino acids, supporting muscle repair, immune function, and overall health. All animal protein sources offer all amino acids.

Chapter 4 Goals:

Nutrition:

Remember, in each chapter, we are building off the last, so try to keep aiming to eat proper serving sizes and 45 grams of carbohydrates per meal of which 7-10 grams are fiber!

For this chapter, your goal is to have protein with every meal and snack, remembering that plant sources and animal sources both count! Remember those plants will also help you reach your fiber goals—the proverbial killing two birds with one stone.

Fitness

Be sure to stretch and walk 10 minutes a day.

Hydration

We are boosting our hydration goal in this chapter; the challenge is to drink 8 ounces when you get up in the morning, 8 ounces in between breakfast and lunch, and 8 ounces in between lunch and dinner.

Red Lentil Curry

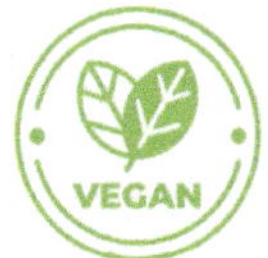

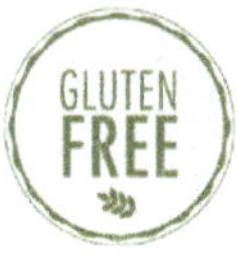

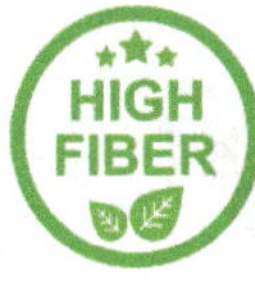

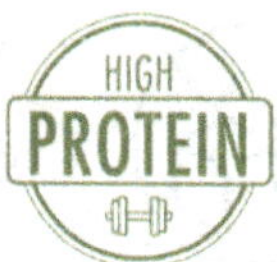

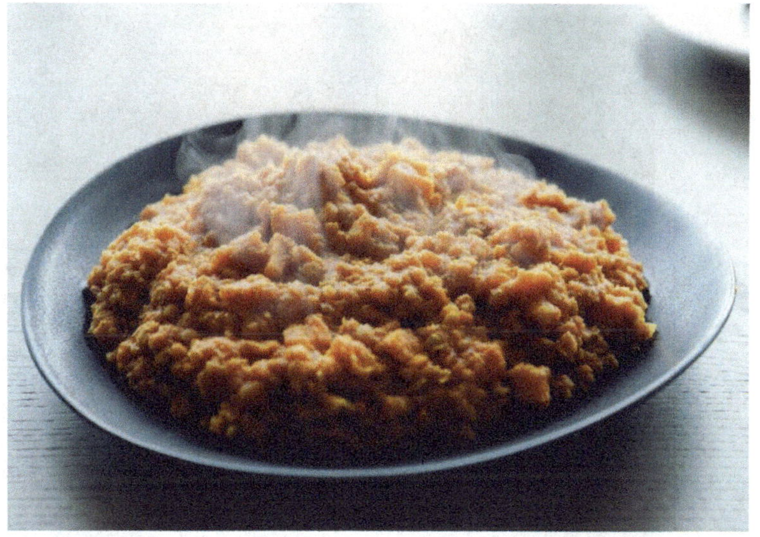

Ingredients

- 2 cups red lentils
- 2 cups sweet potatoes, cubed
- 3/4 cups white onion, chopped
- 2 tsp. Garam masala
- 2 tsp. turmeric
- 2 tsp. fresh ginger, grated
- 3 tsp. garlic, minced
- 3 tsp. Thai red curry paste
- 6 oz. tomato paste
- 3 cups water
- 2 cups vegetable stock, low sodium
- 1 can light coconut milk
- Juice from 1 lemon

Garnish: cilantro or green onions

Directions

Combine all ingredients, except lemon and garnishes, in a Crockpot or Instapot. Stir ingredients to combine and cook on low for 5-6 hours or high for 3-4. Drizzle lemon into mixture. Serve with a gluten-free or whole grain roll of choice, such as brown rice or wild rice, and vegetables, such as broccoli or cauliflower. Garnish with cilantro or green onion. Enjoy warm.

Maple Apple Turkey Burgers

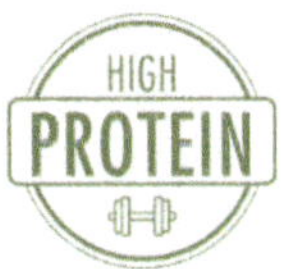

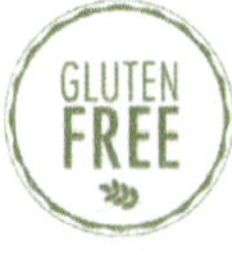

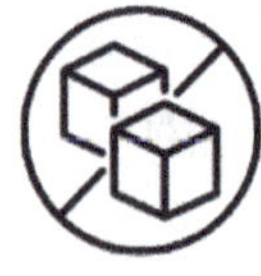

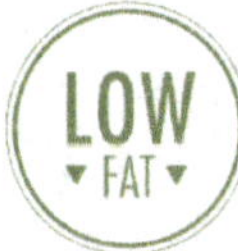

Recipe makes 4 burgers

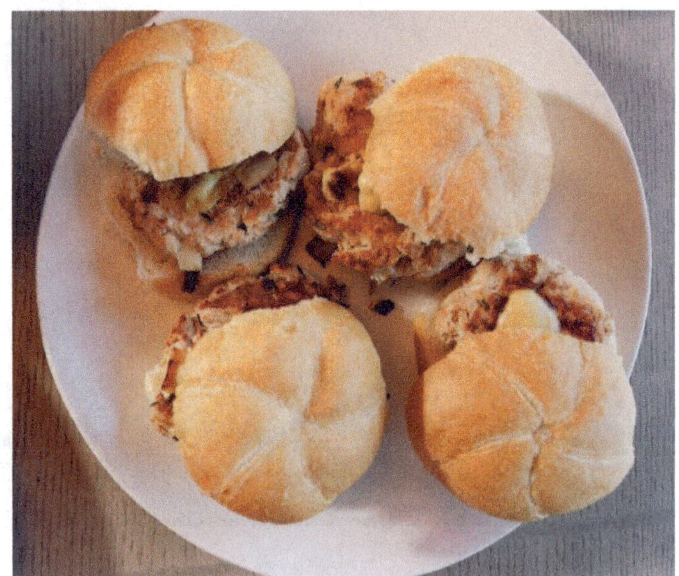

Ingredients

- 1 lb. lean ground turkey
- 1 cup finely chopped granny smith and/or gala apples
- 1/4 tsp. garlic powder
- 1/4 tsp. salt
- 1/4 tsp. paprika
- 1 Tbsp. maple syrup
- 1/4 tsp. fresh rosemary, chopped
- 1/4 tsp. freshly ground black pepper

Directions

Mix spices, apples, and maple syrup into ground turkey and form into 4 burgers.
Fire up the grill or a grill pan to a medium-high heat. Cook on one side for 5-7 minutes.
Flip and cook on the other side another 4-5 minutes or if a meat thermometer reads 165 degrees F.
Serve with choice of toppings on a gluten-free or whole grain roll.
Enjoy!

CHAPTER 5: GETTING THE FACTS ABOUT FAT

I'm going to kick off this chapter with some time travel. That's right; we're going to rewind time back to the early 1990s. Nirvana and alternative rock were taking over radio stations...and the words *fat free* were on food packaging everywhere! One of the most famous brands was Snackwells® cookies. I can taste them now...their Devil's Food Cake cookies were all the talk among young women like myself.

"Fat free" became a trend after a 1988 Surgeon General's Report[xxi] indicated that reducing fat intake should be Americans' number-one priority to reduce the risk of weight gain, heart disease, and cancer. How is it that in this fat-free era, type-2 diabetes and obesity (both precursors and indicators of heart disease) began skyrocketing?

Turns out they were wrong! Research came out in the early 2000s, suggesting that the low-fat trend was making Americans obese and was not lowering the risk of disease. One of the largest studies to compare the long-term effect of going low-fat was published in the Journal of the American Medical Association in 2006.[xxii] Researchers found that low-fat interventions did not reduce the risk of cancer and cardiovascular disease. In 2015, all this research was combined in a meta-analysis, including 53 studies and over 68,000 participants; this meta-analysis concluded that low-fat diets did not result in weight loss.[xxiii]

One of the main reasons why this fat-free trend did not work is because it resulted in people eating more sugar and refined carbohydrates! Some fat is needed in your diet and can help with long-term weight loss and disease prevention. I want you to think of fats as a giant umbrella. Underneath the umbrella, there are good fats and not-so-good fats.

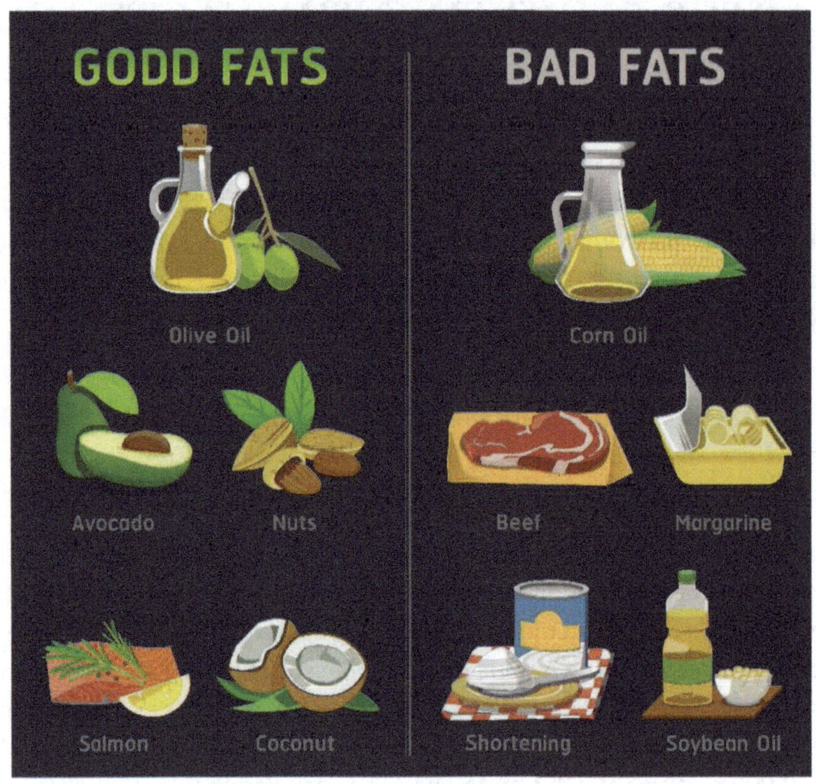

The good fats are unsaturated fats. These fats help lower your LDL cholesterol. These fats come from fish and plants. These types of fats are liquid at room temperature; examples include olive oil, canola oil, and avocado.

Good fats help you absorb vitamins A, D, E, and K. They are called fat-soluble vitamins. When patients come to me with deficiencies in any of these vitamins, I almost always find that they are not consuming enough unsaturated fat.

My patient Susan is in her late 30s. She came to me bewildered by the fact that she was just diagnosed with osteoporosis.

"I'm too young to have this, aren't I?"

It was time for us to investigate why this could be. I had her keep a food journal. After a few entries, I immediately knew what was wrong—she had virtually no unsaturated fat in her diet.

In order to have healthy bone density, not only do you need calcium, magnesium, and other minerals, but also you need vitamin D and K. Vitamin D and K are both fat-soluble vitamins. What this means is that you need unsaturated fat to encapsulate vitamin D and K for your system to absorb them.

Susan was deficient in vitamin D and K. We started adding healthy fats into her diet, and within weeks, she was no longer deficient in these critical vitamins. She also had far less joint pain!

The other side of the umbrella are the not-so-great fats for you. These are saturated fats and trans fats.

Saturated fats come from animal sources and processed and packaged foods For example, say you are having a ribeye steak and see all the marbling; that's saturated fat—something you want to limit (notice I did not say you have to eliminate it).

As for trans fats, these are the fats that you want to avoid at all costs. Trans fats are directly correlated to heart disease. These can be found in foods such as packaged and fried foods.

Trans Fats Explained

So how do you avoid trans fats?

Look at your food labels. There is a section in the label that will list the amount of trans fat.

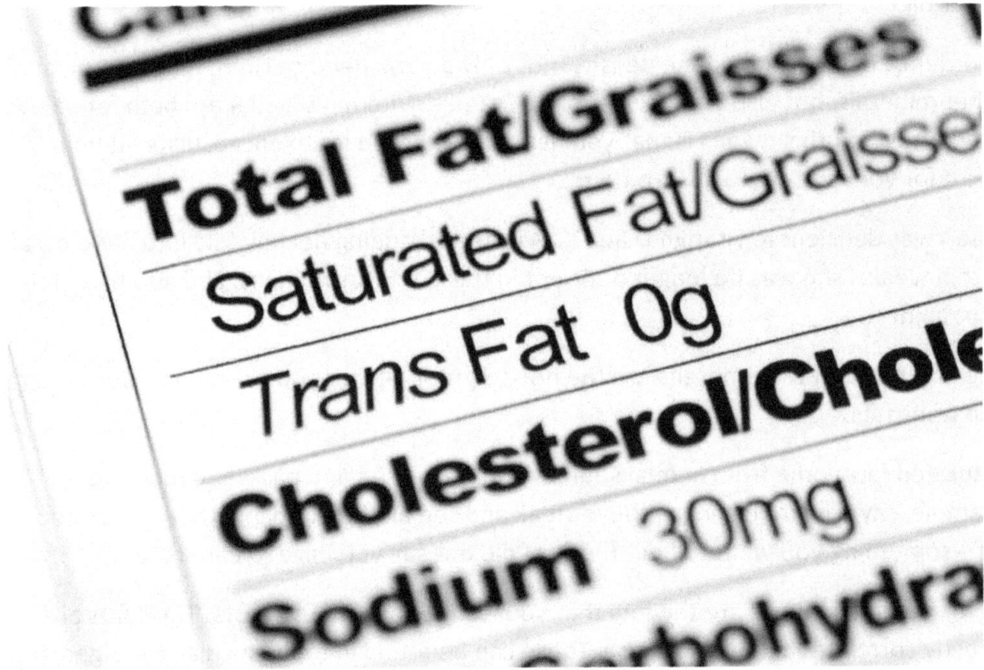

Hopefully, you won't find it often.

In January 2006, the FDA required the food industry to declare the amount of trans fat in food on the Nutrition Facts label. Before then, food companies were not required to list their trans fats. One of the main trans fats you would see in packaged food at the time was partially-hydrogenated oils (PHOs).

After extensive research, the FDA found that PHOs increase your risk of developing heart disease. They felt that by eliminating trans fats from packaged foods, thousands of heart attacks could be prevented each year.[xxiv]

FDA has taken steps to remove artificial trans fats in processed foods. In 2015, FDA determined that PHOs, the major source of artificial trans fats in the food supply, are no longer "Generally Recognized as Safe," or GRAS.

Unfortunately, many packaged foods still contain PHOs like coffee creamer and packaged baked goods.

The other culprits of trans fats are fried food and baked goods.

Fried food is loaded with trans fats, which is a big reason I recommend patients to use air fryers for foods they typically like deep fried like chicken wings and French fries. They taste just as good, but don't contain the trans fats Give it a try!

A Glimpse at Smoke Points

What a lot of people do not know is that if you take a beautiful, wonderful, healthy unsaturated fat like olive oil and you fry it to the point of smoking, you are creating a trans fat! This is called a smoke point.

Never heard of a smoke point? It's just like what it sounds like. It's taking oil and cooking it at a temperature where it begins to smoke.

Smoke Point Heat Levels

Oil Type	Heat
Coconut	High
Avocado	High
Sunflower	High
Safflower	High
Peanut	High
Sesame	Medium
Extra Virgin Olive	Medium
Hazelnut	Medium
Macadamia Nut	Medium
Any Unrefined Oil	Low
Hemp Seed	Low

You want to make sure you are using the right type of oil for the right type of cooking. This chart shows you the smoke point all types of oils. As you can see, these vary in temperatures they can withstand before smoking.

What this chart is showing you is that there are different types of oil you are going to want to use for different cooking methods. For instance, olive oil is great for dipping, salads, and low temperature cooking versus avocado oil, which has a very high smoke point, so it is a good choice when making a stir-fry at a high temperature.

When you cook with the right oils, the added advantage is that you won't smoke out your house!

Fat Density

While I am recommending healthy fats, you still need to be careful not to eat too much fat because it is very calorie-dense.

I will never encourage counting calories, but I am going to show you a little calculation to hopefully shed some light on fats.

To determine how many calories are in fat, you multiple the grams of fat by 9.

To determine how many calories are in protein, you multiply the grams of protein by 4.

And carbohydrate calories are measured the same way that protein is, you multiply the grams of carbs by 4.

Let me share with you a surprising example of how fat soars the calories of a meal to the sky!

I was in New York City when they started listing calories on menus. I was at a generic restaurant and was ready to order a Cobb salad and noticed that it had 1,200 calories while a burger only had 700 calories. This may be perplexing right? The reason why the Cobb salad had so many calories is because it had FIVE fat sources: egg, bacon, avocado, cheese, and dressing!

We need fat in our diet; we should just be mindful about how much fat is in our meals.

Let's break down this salad by determining which ingredients are unsaturated fats and which are saturated.

The unsaturated fats are the oil-based dressing and the avocado, while the saturated fats are the cheese, bacon, and egg yolk (the yummy stuff). I'm not saying to never have those yummy ingredients, but having these ingredients together is too much.

All About Omegas (PUFAs and MUFAs):

Omega-3s, Omega-6s, and Omega-9s are essential fatty acids. Your body doesn't have the enzymes to produce them, so you must get them from your diet. Omega-3s and Omega-6s are what we call PUFAs, short for polyunsaturated fatty acids and Omega-9s are MUFAS, short for monounsaturated fatty acids.

You can get Omega-3 essential fatty acids by eating fish twice a week as recommended by the American Heart Association.[xxv] The best fish sources of Omega-3s are tuna and salmon. If you do not like the taste of seafood, you can take fish oil capsules that are flavored with lemon to disguise the fish taste. Vegans can get their Omega-3s from hemp seeds, chia seeds, flax seeds, and walnuts.

There are also Omega-6 fatty acids. These come from all sorts of vegetable oils. Keep in mind, a lot of packaged foods use these oils. Omega-6s are pro-inflammatory. You do need some inflammation in your body, because inflammation works to repair tissue damage, kill off harmful invaders, and restore balance to your body. Without inflammation, you wouldn't be able to heal from injuries or fight off infections effectively.

However, too much inflammation is the precursor to all chronic ailments from obesity to heart disease, from arthritis to Alzheimer's.

It is so important to get enough Omega-3s in your diet to offset the amount of Omega-6s you are consuming.

If you rewind time back to the period when humans were just evolving, there wasn't such an imbalance of Omega-6s to Omega-3s. The ratio then was 1:1. One-hundred years ago, the ratio of Omega 3s to Omega-6s to Omega-3s was between 2:1 to 4:1. Over time, this ratio has become higher and higher because of the amount of food processed with oils high in Omega-6s. Today, the ratio is 20:1 in most Americans or even higher.[xxvi]

Diving Deeper into Omega-3s and Omega-6s

It can get confusing because Omegas are considered "essential," yet we must be careful we don't consume too much Omega-6! Yep, that's true. But I am here to guide you.

The three Omega-3s include (these are the 3 amino acids!) ALA (alpha-linolenic acid), DHA (docosahexaenoic acid), and EPA (eicosatetraenoic acid). ALA is primarily found in plants, while DHA and EPA are found in animal sources and algae.

ALA is likely the most common Omega-3 in your diet. This Omega-3 gives you energy. It can be found in avocados, whole wheat bread, oats, navy beans, chia seeds, walnuts, flaxseeds, canola oil, hemp seeds, and soybeans. Some ALA converts into EPA and DHA as well.

EPA is essential for heart health and can reduce your triglyceride (fat in the blood) levels and your blood pressure. EPA is found in fatty fish such as tuna and salmon. It is also found in eggs.

DHA is so important because it comprises the gray matter in your brain, keeping you sharp and helping you to focus. It can also help protect you from dementia and Alzheimer's. Foods that are high in DHA are essentially the same foods that have high amounts of EPA.

Now let's get into the sneaky Omega-6s and why we do need *some* Omega-6s in our diets. The two main Omega-6 fatty acids are arachidonic and linoleic acid. Sources of linoleic acid include vegetable oils, nuts, and seeds; arachidonic acid is found in meat and eggs.

Both Omega-6s help with heart health, but too much can cause inflammation. The best way to reduce your Omega-6s and improve your Omega-6: Omega-3 ratio is to reduce the consumption of packaged foods that are made with oils very high in Omega-6, including: corn, cottonseed, soybean, and sunflower seed oils. Also, another way to be mindful of keeping your ratio balanced is to avoid using these oils in your cooking.

MUFAs

MUFA, or monounsaturated fat, is another healthy fat. The most common form of MUFA in our diets comes from oleic acid, which is a type of Omega-9 Fatty Acid. Oleic acid can be made by the body, but it also can be found in foods. The highest levels are found in olive oil.

A recent meta-analysis published in the peer-reviewed journal, *Advances in Nutrition*,[xxvii] reviewed several studies on oleic acid-enriched diets, finding that the subjects lost substantial weight and also reduced their belly fat, decreasing their risk of type diabetes, heart disease, osteoarthritis, and other chronic diseases. Scientists have also discovered that oleic acid can help reduce blood pressure, again decreasing your risk of heart disease.

Olive oil, avocados, peanuts, and peanut butter all have Omega-9s. These are great for improving your cholesterol levels when eaten in moderation and especially when replacing saturated fat with them. For example, using avocado oil in your cooking instead of corn oil.

When it comes to fat consumption, individuals taking GLP-1 medications need to make sure they are getting sufficient unsaturated fat for all the benefits. And they should be incredibly careful about the amount of saturated and trans fat they consume. In an interview with Dr. Robert Gabbay, Chief Scientific and Medical Officer of the American Diabetes Association, he said, "avoiding high-fat food is also critical, because they can make people taking [GLP-1 medications] feel uncomfortably, even painfully full."[xxviii]

Confusing Cholesterol and Triglycerides

We cannot talk about fat without talking about cholesterol and triglycerides, which are both types of lipids (fats) in your blood.

Growing up, my mom always watched labels, trying to avoid anything that was high in cholesterol.

When I first learned about cholesterol twenty years and up until very recently, LDL was considered bad and "Lousy," and HDL was touted as being good and "Happy."

Avoiding cholesterol from food and calling LDL the bad guy are inaccurate approaches.

You need cholesterol to produce estrogen and testosterone and to absorb vitamin D from sunshine!

What we now know is that LDL cholesterol is NOT bad. When we consume cholesterol from food, our liver will make less. The problem is not the cholesterol levels you see on the labels; it's the Standard American Diet in general, which is loaded with inflammatory foods—foods that are high in simple carbohydrates, sugar, and both saturated and trans fats.

Imagine that inflammation causes the liver to send out an LDL cholesterol dump truck to drop LDL off at inflammation sites.

If we didn't have inflammation, we'd naturally have lower LDL cholesterol levels.

When we have a high LDL level, we have inflammation. So, if you reduce your intake of the foods that cause inflammation, you'll reduce your LDL.

A diet high in inflammatory foods leads to type-2 diabetes, high blood pressure, and hyperlipidemia (high cholesterol).

Taking cholesterol-lowering medications may help, but just as nutrition can help improve health for those taking GLP-1 medication, it can do the same for those taking medications to lower cholesterol.

If you do take cholesterol-lowering medication, it can interfere with vitamin D and estrogen production, which could ultimately lead to osteoporosis. Be sure your medical provider is monitoring your vitamin D and estrogen levels.

Think back to my favorite f-word from the carbohydrates chapter—fiber! When we consume fiber sources, the resulting healthy bacteria in our gut signals the liver to produce HDL cholesterol. Think of HDL cholesterol as front loaders. The liver sends out HDL front loaders to pick up the LDL cholesterol and filter it out of the body.

Foods high in fiber also have plant sterols.

Plant sterols have the same molecular makeup as cholesterol. Your body will uptake the plant sterols before up taking cholesterol.

You can consume plenty of plant sterols from whole grains, plant-based proteins, and fruits and vegetables.

Isn't it great news that you can reverse high cholesterol, type-2 diabetes, and most chronic conditions through diet?

Nutrition is everything. Simple changes will make a huge difference.

You can also increase your HDL cholesterol by increasing daily exercise. When you exercise, your liver produces more HDL cholesterol.

I can't end my discussion about cholesterol without sharing my own testimony. I was working at Wegmans as their dietitian, and we had someone come in to give free biometric screenings. The nurse pricked my finger and told me "You have high cholesterol."

Laughing, I told her, "There is NO way. I am a dietitian, and I walk my talk."

I went to see my doctor the following week and sure enough I had high cholesterol. I evaluated my diet—too much partaking in charcuterie boards. I had to change my ways and switched to low-fat cheese and made sure my protein sources were most often either from lean meats or were plant-based.

Six months later, I had a checkup and was happily flabbergasted to learn that my cholesterol dropped 60 points!

This inspired me to experiment some more. You know that egg debate you hear all the time in the media? One month, eggs are good for you; the next month, they are bad for you. I had to settle this once and for all.

I love eggs; I started eating 2-3 every morning. And guess what? I had NO increase in my cholesterol! This is where the topic of cholesterol can be tricky. I have had patients avoid eggs because they are high in cholesterol just like my mom used to do. The thing is that the dietary cholesterol in eggs does not affect your total cholesterol. The dietary benefits of eggs far outweigh any fat. Eggs are loaded with iodine, vitamin D, vitamin E, and amazing protein!

So, let's talk about cholesterol lab work. If you get your cholesterol checked and your total cholesterol is high, don't freak out yet! If your HDL is high and your LDL is low, that's okay—you are in good health. If your LDL is high and your HDL is low; that's when you need to focus on making nutritional changes like those mentioned throughout this book. It's better to have high cholesterol with a high HDL than it would be to have a normal cholesterol level with a low HDL. If your overall cholesterol level is high but your HDL levels are also high, it may offset some of the risks associated with high cholesterol levels.

Triglycerides are another type of lipid that doctors often order alongside cholesterol lab work. Triglycerides are an essential source of energy for the body. When you eat, your body converts any calories it doesn't need to use right away into triglycerides. These triglycerides are stored in fat cells and released later when your body needs energy between meals. They're particularly important for providing energy to muscles.

However, having high triglyceride levels (200 mg/dL or above) is a concern because it can contribute to the buildup of fatty deposits in artery walls. This increases your risk of heart disease.

Chapter 5 Summary:

- The chapter begins with a nostalgic trip back to the early 1990s, highlighting the prevalence of the "fat-free" trend, epitomized by brands like Snackwells cookies.

- Despite the Surgeon General's 1988 report advocating for reduced fat intake to combat weight gain and heart disease, subsequent research in the early 2000s revealed that low-fat diets were not effective and may have contributed to obesity and type-2 diabetes.

- A significant study published in the *Journal of the American Medical Association* in 2006 found that low-fat interventions did not reduce the risk of cancer and cardiovascular disease.

- The chapter emphasizes the importance of distinguishing between good fats (unsaturated fats) and harmful fats (saturated and trans fats).

- Unsaturated fats, found in olive oil, canola oil, and avocado, are crucial for absorbing fat-soluble vitamins like A, D, E, and K, as illustrated by a patient's experience with osteoporosis due to a lack of unsaturated fat in her diet.

- Saturated fats, mainly from animal sources and processed/packaged foods, should be limited, while trans fats, correlated with heart disease, should be avoided altogether by checking food labels for partially hydrogenated oils (PHOs).

- The concept of smoke points is introduced, emphasizing the importance of using the right type of oil for different cooking methods to avoid creating trans fats.

- Omega-3 and Omega-6 fatty acids (PUFAS), essential for health but needing a balanced intake, are discussed, with emphasis on sources like fish, nuts, and seeds.

- Monounsaturated fats (MUFAs) from sources like olive oil and avocados are highlighted as beneficial for cholesterol levels.

- Individuals taking GLP-1 receptor agonists are advised to be careful about their saturated fat and trans fat intake, as high-fat foods can cause discomfort and even pain for these individuals, according to Dr. Robert Gabbay, Chief Scientific and Medical Officer of the American Diabetes Association.

Chapter 5 Goals:

As always, you are going to continue goals from the previous chapters and build on them.

Nutrition: Continue to be mindful of serving sizes. Ensure that you are consuming enough fiber and lean protein. Starting now, make sure you have some healthy fat at each meal.

Also, don't forget to continue your food journal!

Fitness: Let's increase the walking to 15 minutes a day—and continue to stretch.

Hydration: You are going to increase your hydration each chapter—and trust me, it will get easier and easier. Try having 8 ounces of water as soon as you wake up. Then, drink 8 ounces at breakfast, 16 ounces between breakfast and lunch, and another 8 ounces between lunch and dinner. This adds up to a total of 40 ounces.

Avocado Toast with Egg and Spinach

Recipe makes one individual serving

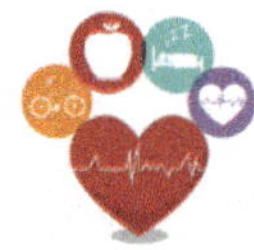
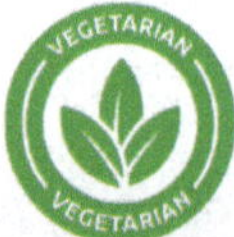

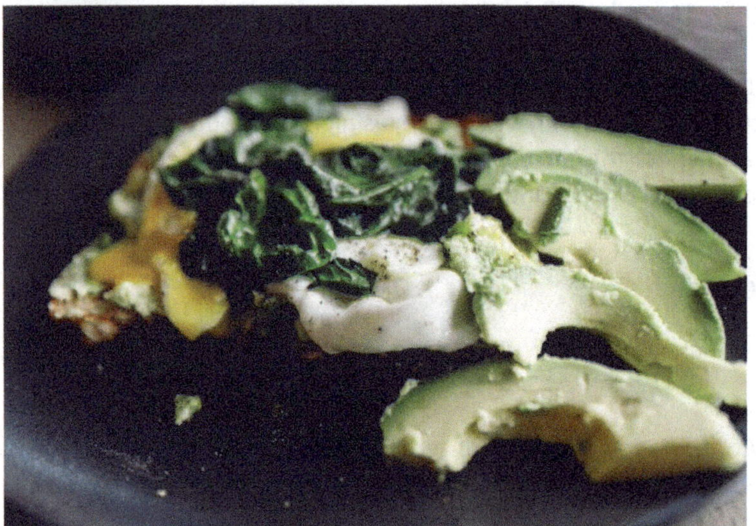

Ingredients

- One half of an avocado
- 1 egg
- 1 slice of whole grain bread, toasted
- 1/2 cup spinach
- Seasoning of your choice
- 1 Tbsp. of avocado oil

Directions

Place a medium sized pan on medium to low heat. Add avocado oil to the pan and heat up. Once the pan is heated, crack the egg into the pan. While the egg is cooking, scoop the avocado into the bowl, mash up and add seasonings of your choice into the avocado. Place a slice of whole grain bread in the toaster or oven. Cook the egg for 2-3 minutes. While egg is cooking, scoop and spread avocado on toast. Flip the egg over and cook for 20-30 seconds. Place the over easy egg on the toasted bread and seasoned avocado. Place the spinach in the pan and cook until wilted and then place on top of the egg.

**This recipe is very customizable, switching up the leafy green and type of seasoning of your choice!

Lemon Garlic Salmon
Recipe makes 2 servings

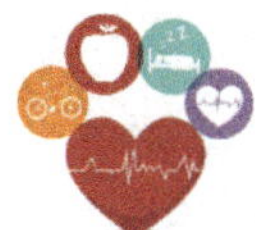
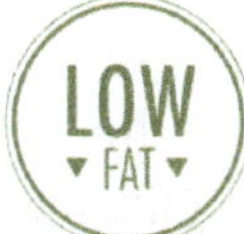

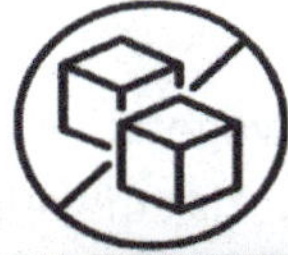
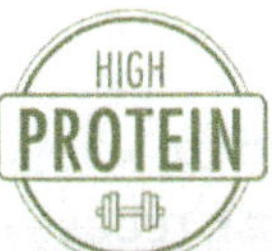

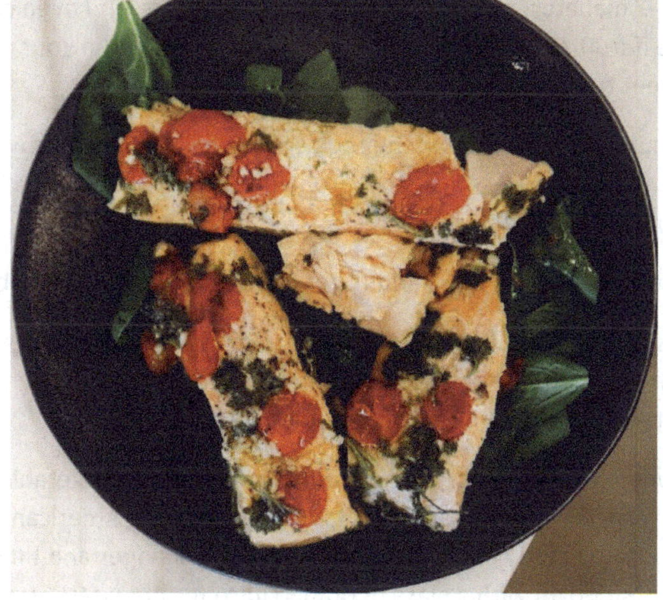

Ingredients

- Aluminum foil
- 1/2 lb. fresh salmon filets, divided into two portions
- 1 cup cherry tomatoes
- 2 Tbsp. olive oil
- 2 Tbsp. honey
- 2 Tbsp. lemon juice
- 2 garlic cloves, minced
- 2 Tbsp. fresh parsley, chopped

Directions

Preheat oven to 400 degrees F. Lay out 2 sheets of aluminum foil, large enough to surround salmon and leave space. In a small bowl, mix olive oil, honey, lemon juice, parsley and garlic. Place salmon and cherry tomatoes on foil and pour mixture on top of each filet. Wrap aluminum foil around salmon and seal tightly. Bake 20-25 minutes. Transfer contents of aluminum foil to a plate, discard foil. Enjoy!

CHAPTER 6: FALLING IN LOVE WITH FRUITS AND VEGGIES

Your mom was right when she said to "eat your vegetables", and the same goes for fruit. Eating fruit and vegetables can reduce your risk of weight gain, high blood pressure, type-2 diabetes, stroke, heart disease, vision loss, and even cancer.[xxix] This is especially true if fruit and vegetables replace unhealthy foods in your diet, such as salty snacks and sweet treats.

Take, for example, my patient John; he replaced his daily candy bars with a piece of fruit. He has more energy, less digestive problems, and he is helping to protect himself from dozens of chronic diseases.

But did you know that only 1 in 10 adults get enough fruits and vegetables every day?[xxx]

This statistic is staggering to me. Despite encouragement from parents to eat vegetables and even learning the importance of fruit and vegetables in school, why are 90% of Americans not getting enough fruits and vegetables?

The reasons why are complex. A recent study[xxxi] showed that vegetable consumption decreased because the number one vegetable eaten among Americans (potatoes) decreased. This same study pointed out that "lifestyle changes and time constraints can determine if we sit down with a glass of orange juice for breakfast, grab a banana on the way out, or forgo the meal altogether. Time for and interest in cooking play a role, too...The price of products and the income available to buy them can also affect a person's food choices."

My number one goal as a dietitian is to get people to eat more fruits and vegetables. If you don't do anything else, at least do this!

Because of the appetite reduction that takes place when taking GLP-1 medications, it may be hard to meet your daily requirement of fruits and veggies. Make it a point to fit them in!

I have had several patients use time and money as reasons why they don't eat many fruits or vegetables. If you eat in-season or eat frozen or canned fruits and vegetables, I promise you that it won't be as expensive as you think.

Others have expressed concern over not eating organic. They stray away from what the Environmental Working Group calls the Dirty Dozen[xxxii] because they are afraid of pesticide exposure.

But trust me, eating those nonorganic supposed dirty dozen fruits and veggies (like kale and strawberries) is way better than not eating them at all. You will not be consuming enough pesticides to harm you.

In fact, Carl Winter, a toxicologist, investigated the pesticide levels of the Dirty Dozen list and found that if a person truly ate the 12 "dirty" foods on the list regularly, the exposure to most of the pesticides would be less than 0.01% of the chronic exposure level that the Environmental Protection Agency (EPA) considers possibly harmful.[xxxiii]

Fruits and vegetables are so awesome because they are low in calories yet high in fiber, vitamins, minerals, and nutrients! All fruits and vegetables are "super foods."

Let's dive deep into the *why* and *how* fruits and vegetables are so protective, how much you should have, and fun ways to incorporate them into your daily lives.

Antioxidants

One of the most amazing qualities about fruits and vegetables is the fact that they boast a ton of antioxidants. You may be thinking, I see that word, "antioxidants," all the time, but I have no idea what it means. It is a buzz word—you may see it on everything from food to face lotion.

Let's break down the role of antioxidants. Antioxidants help neutralize free radicals in your body. Free radicals are not good; they come from stress, poor diet, smoking, excessive exercise. They can even come from living and breathing in the air around you. Free radicals cause inflammation, which contributes to all the chronic diseases I mentioned above. Antioxidants give free radicals electrons so that they cannot cause havoc in the body.

Three major antioxidants that I want to highlight are vitamins A, C, and E. Think of these antioxidants as scavengers/scrapers of free radicals. They scrape up these free radicals, and then imagine that these awesome antioxidants add these awful free radicals to a train car—you have the vitamin A car, the vitamin C car, the vitamin E car and so on. You need all of these to neutralize free radicals and drive them on this train, right out of your body!

Your body does not produce these antioxidants, so you need to get them from food!

The way you get vitamin A from vegetables and fruit is through beta carotene; this is usually found in yellow and orange fruits and vegetables (carrots, sweet potatoes, pumpkins, cantaloupe, mangoes). Beta carotene converts to vitamin A in your digestive tract (cool, right?). Vitamin A is known for helping vision and has also been shown to help prevent metabolic syndrome and help keep triglyceride levels at a healthy level.

Vitamin C comes from a wide array of fruits and vegetables. Did you know that eating five large strawberries is 100% of the vitamin C you need for a day? Citrus fruits, cruciferous vegetables (broccoli, cabbage, cauliflower), and leafy greens are all very powerful sources of vitamin C as well.

Did you know that vitamin C deficiency was responsible for scurvy, a painful disease, that killed millions of sailors between the 16th and 18th centuries? A British doctor realized that the sailors that consumed lime juice (one of the few fresh fruits that could survive long sailing journeys) did not contract scurvy. They were getting enough vitamin C antioxidants to protect them from the disease! These sailors were coined the name "limeys."

Not only can vitamin C bolster your immune system, but also it helps form collagen; it helps you to absorb iron; it also aids in maintaining cartilage, bones, and teeth.

Vitamin E is found in leafy greens (also in nuts), and it is very beneficial to the health of your brain, blood, and skin.

It's important that I mention that vitamin A and vitamin E are both fat-soluble antioxidants. As I mentioned in the last chapter, you need good, healthy fat sources to be able to absorb fat-soluble vitamins like A and E.

Each color of fruit or vegetable represents a different antioxidant. These antioxidants will combat the effects of free radicals. Getting all colors of fruits and vegetables will ensure that you have all the cars on the train needed to neutralize the free radicals and reduce inflammation.

Antioxidants are the best thing for your body! The bonus is they can help keep you looking youthful for years. Save yourself some money—instead of buying creams and serums boasting about their antioxidants, you can get these by eating your fruits and veggies!

Let me tell you about some fruits and veggies that are super loaded with antioxidants.

Blueberries

All berries are high in antioxidants, but I'd like to pay special attention to blueberries. Can you believe those tiny berries are packed with antioxidants? Several studies have even suggested that blueberries have more antioxidants than any fruit or vegetable![xxxiv][xxxv] *WebMD* says this about blueberries: "Just one cup has 13,427 total antioxidants—vitamins A and C, plus flavonoids (a type of antioxidant) like quercetin and anthocyanidin. That's about 10 times the USDA's recommendation, in just one cup!"

Blueberries (and all berries) are great choices for people taking GLP-1 medications because they are lower in sugar than most fruits. It is imperative for individuals with type-2 diabetes, including those taking GLP-1 medications, to watch their sugar consumption.

Kale

There is a reason that kale has become a "trendy" veggie—this cruciferous veggie is loaded with antioxidants. It is high in vitamin C and beta carotene. It is also high in antioxidants called quercetin and kaempferol, both of which help promote heart health and protect your nervous system.[xxxvi]

All Red Fruits and Veggies

I highly recommend tomatoes, red onions, red bell peppers, papaya, watermelon, and all pink and red veggies. They are high in vitamin C and A and they have an antioxidant called lycopene, which reduces your risk of diabetes, heart disease, and cancer. Like vitamin A and E, research studies[xxxvii] have found that you can absorb more lycopene with healthy fats. For example, if you add a little bit of olive oil to your tomato sauce, you will likely absorb more of the lycopene from the tomatoes.

Fruit and Veggie Synergy

Like the tomato and olive oil example, there are several examples of food synergy—how combining one type of food with another can help you absorb a certain nutrient. Here are some of my favorite examples from the fruits and vegetables categories. Consider these pairs of food as collaborators:

-Tomatoes and Spinach

Spinach is a good source of iron, and the tomatoes have quite a bit of vitamin C; the vitamin C in the tomatoes helps your body to absorb the iron in the spinach.

-Lemon and Kale

The vitamin C in lemon helps you to absorb the iron in kale. Lemon adds a lot of flavor to leafy greens too!

-Black Beans and Red Bell Peppers

The vitamin C in red bell peppers can enhance the absorption of nonheme iron from plant-based sources like black beans, making it a great combination for vegetarians.

-Berries and Dark Chocolate

The flavonoids in dark chocolate can enhance the absorption of antioxidants from berries, creating a delicious and nutritious dessert.

-Chard and Oranges

The vitamin C in oranges can improve the absorption of iron from Swiss chard, making it a nutritious combination for salads and side dishes.

-Salad Greens and Nuts

Adding nuts to your salad provides healthy fats and protein that can enhance the absorption of fat-soluble vitamins found in leafy greens.

-Carrots and Avocado

Carrots have beta carotene, turning into vitamin A, which is fat soluble. The healthy fats from avocado help you to absorb the beta carotene. Consider tossing both in a salad.

-Bok Choy and Salmon

Bok choy is loaded with calcium while salmon is a good source of vitamin D. Vitamin D helps you to absorb calcium.

Portion Size

One thing that many of my patients have been confused about is a good portion size for fruits and vegetables. It depends on the carbohydrates in each choice.

Fruits are considered carbohydrates. They contain a naturally-occurring sugar called fructose. Some have more than others. For example, a good serving of fruit would be an entire cup of berries, a half of banana, or a medium-sized apple. While the fruit has carbs; keep in mind that they have fiber too. You can refer back to pages 31-32 for the fiber content of different fruits. You should have 2-3 servings of fruit a day.

I once had this patient from Italy who couldn't understand why she was gaining weight when she was eating everything healthy; come to find out, she was eating about four servings of fruit with most meals. That is too much! We swapped out some of her fruit for vegetables and added in a little protein; she was able to lose 30 pounds and keep it off!

Be careful with dried fruit. When I talk about dried fruit, I am reminded of a college lacrosse player that came to speak to me at a talk I gave at Hobart and William Smith College. She was so enthusiastic and shared with me that she ate an entire bag of dried mangoes almost every day. I looked at the bag and that would equal about 160 grams of sugar. Dried fruits and vegetables are great—but a serving size is only 1-2 tablespoons. During the drying process, the water decreases and the natural sugars in the fruit become more concentrated. This means that dried fruit ends up with a higher sugar content per volume compared to fresh fruit.

You can have more vegetables than fruit. I like to see half the plate as vegetables.

I do need to address the difference between starchy veggies and non starchy veggies. The starchy veggies (potatoes, acorn squash, butternut squash, peas, corn, sweet potatoes) are high in carbohydrates, which will turn into glucose. Too much of these can spike your blood sugar.

Non starchy veggies are higher in fiber and have fewer calories than starchy veggies. There are hundreds of choices here. Some of my favorites are olives, eggplant, broccoli, cabbage, tomatoes, red peppers, zucchini, arugula, brussels sprouts.

Both starchy and non starchy veggies are high in nutrients. Just keep in mind to have both types. I have had many patients whose veggies with dinner only ever consisted of potatoes or corn.

I challenge you to eat three new veggies every week. We get into these habits of eating the same ol' veggies all the time. Change them up. Try something new. Get all the colors of the rainbow!

Hot and Cold Vegetables

A helpful tip to get more veggies in at dinner is to have one hot vegetable and one cold vegetable. For example, you can have some raw carrots with a little bit of ranch dip and some hot Brussel sprouts or maybe a salad with some steamed green beans. This keeps your meals interesting instead of filling a half plate with just one vegetable like broccoli.

Frozen Fruits and Veggies

Keep frozen fruits and vegetables on hand; this is a great way to ensure that you have veggies for your meals. Frozen fruits and vegetables are picked at their peak and immediately frozen, keeping all the nutrients intact. Frozen fruits and veggies are cheaper too, especially when the fresh fruits and vegetables are out of season!

Another bonus of frozen veggies and fruits is that they can't go bad in your freezer. I can't even count the number of patients that I have had who avoid buying fruits and vegetables because they can never get through them before they go bad. That's not possible when you choose frozen!

Stocking up on "new" veggies can be easy by hitting up the frozen vegetable aisle. You can even count things like riced cauliflower or zucchini noodles.

Canned Fruits and Vegetables

Keep canned fruits and vegetables in your pantry too. These tend to be relatively affordable. Just be sure to rinse them. Veggies may have excess sodium and fruit may have sugary syrup in them. By rinsing them, you can drastically reduce the sodium or sugar content.

Enhance the Flavors of Veggies with Spices

A lot of my patients come to me saying they never liked vegetables. A popular reason why is because so many people grew up with boiled vegetables seasoned with salt and butter.

You are in control of preparing your veggies these days. Try other methods like roasting. For example, my patient Mike never liked brussels sprouts, but he does now! I suggested he chop them in half and season them with a little olive oil and Italian seasoning and then roast them. He can't get enough of them!

You will find many flavorful ways to prepare your veggies in the recipe section of this chapter.

Consider having a piece of fruit before a meal

A recent article published in the *International Journal of Environmental Research and Public Health*, found that "consumption of fruit before a meal was more likely to lead to satiation than after a meal or no fruit."[xxxviii] The researchers concluded that consumption of fruit before a meal suppresses appetite and could potentially help in weight regulation. Enjoying a salad before a meal would likely have the same effect.

Preparing your veggies ahead of time

One easy way to get your veggies is to have them as snacks! It can be fun!

The next time you do your weekly grocery shopping, hit up the produce section and shop the rainbow. For example, get some red, yellow, and green bell peppers, some broccoli and cauliflower, a couple red onions, some mixed greens.

Be realistic—don't buy more fruits and veggies than you and your family will consume. You don't want to waste food. Also visit the frozen section and stock your freezer with frozen fruits and veggies.

Now that you have fruits and veggies at home, do some prep work for the week. Slice up those peppers and shred some carrots so that you can mix them in with a salad. Make a big fruit salad with melons and pineapple. Chop broccoli and cauliflower heads so that they are easy to work with for a busy week-night dinner.

For busy weeks, buy a veggie tray on Sundays and make up little individual bags for each day of the week. I once had a patient who was a teacher, Julia, who did this and lost fifty pounds. I ran into her five years later, and she told me that she was still doing it and kept the weight off.

Some patients have balked at the idea of buying a veggie tray, saying that it would be too expensive, but we did some research and found out that if you bought all the broccoli, cauliflower, tomatoes, celery, carrots, peppers, and radishes and dip separately, it was cheaper buying the tray and you didn't have to cut it up or anything!

Fruits and Veggies Can Be for Breakfast Too

I have had a lot of patients skip breakfast or go for something like a bagel muffin or bowl of cereal. Well, consider some quick and easy options that include veggies or fruit.

I love tossing berries into my morning oatmeal or Greek yogurt and granola. Take some of those sliced peppers, some presliced mushrooms and some onion and sauté them together; add a couple of eggs; and voila you have an omelet.

Dips for Flavor

Experiment with healthy dips like a low-fat ranch or hummus. My patient Michael said, "I never imagined in my life that I would eat hummus, but it is actually really good and there are so many different flavors that I never get bored. Vegetables and hummus has become my favorite snack—way better than potato chips!"

Be Careful with "Juicing" and Smoothies

I get a little nervous when patients tell me they're juicing because while the juice may have vitamins and minerals, that's also where all the sugar goes. And the fiber ends up in the pulp, which is thrown out. You want the fiber to help stabilize those blood-sugar levels.

Some people use a blender, which will keep the fiber in the juice. This is better, but still not ideal. Chewing your food is way better than drinking your food. When you chew your food, you spur your stomach acids to produce the hormones and gut bacteria needed to boost your metabolism.

Also, be careful with smoothies. Smoothies can be healthy for sure, but I want you to think about how much sugar can be in those smoothies. If you include a banana, a cup of berries, yogurt, and apple juice you could end up with way over the amount of carbs you should have in a day. Check out the healthy smoothie recipe I provide at the end of Chapter 12.

Chapter 6 Summary:

- Consuming fruits and vegetables reduces the risk of various diseases such as weight gain, high blood pressure, type-2 diabetes, stroke, heart disease, vision loss, and cancer, especially when replacing unhealthy foods.

- Despite awareness, only 1 in 10 adults meet the daily recommended intake of fruits and vegetables. Factors influencing low consumption include lifestyle changes, time constraints, cooking interests, and economic factors affecting food choices.

- I emphasize increasing fruit and vegetable intake as the number-one goal for better health. It can be hard when taking GLP-1 medications due to appetite reduction, but these are essential to prevent malnutrition.

- Eating in-season, frozen, or canned fruits and vegetables can be cost-effective.

- Fruits and vegetables are rich in antioxidants, such as vitamins A, C, and E, which neutralize harmful free radicals in the body, reducing inflammation and lowering the risk of chronic diseases.

- Combining certain fruits and vegetables enhances the absorption of nutrients, such as pairing tomatoes with olive oil or citrus fruits with leafy greens.

- Watch your serving sizes—especially with canned fruit (one can may have more than 3 servings). Limit dried fruit and be careful with smoothies. Too much can mean too many carbohydrates.

- Experimenting with cooking methods, spices, and healthy dips can make vegetables more appealing, and incorporating fruits and vegetables into breakfast can enhance nutritional intake.

Chapter 6 Goals:

Are you ready to try adding some more fruit and veggies into your day? I hope my tips and the recipes inspire you.

Nutrition: I want to see if you can get a serving of fruit added to each breakfast, and I want you to aim to have a veggie for each meal and snack.

Fitness: Try to do 5-10 squats daily. Imagine you are sitting into a chair and go as low as you can.

Hydration: Try to have at least 32 ounces of water before lunch.

Green Goddess Salad
Serves 8

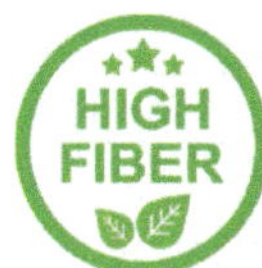

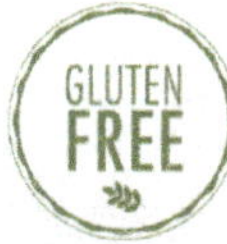

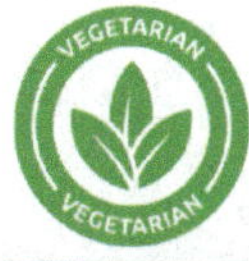

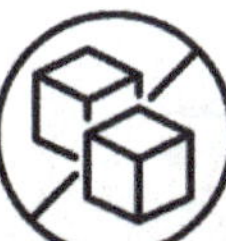

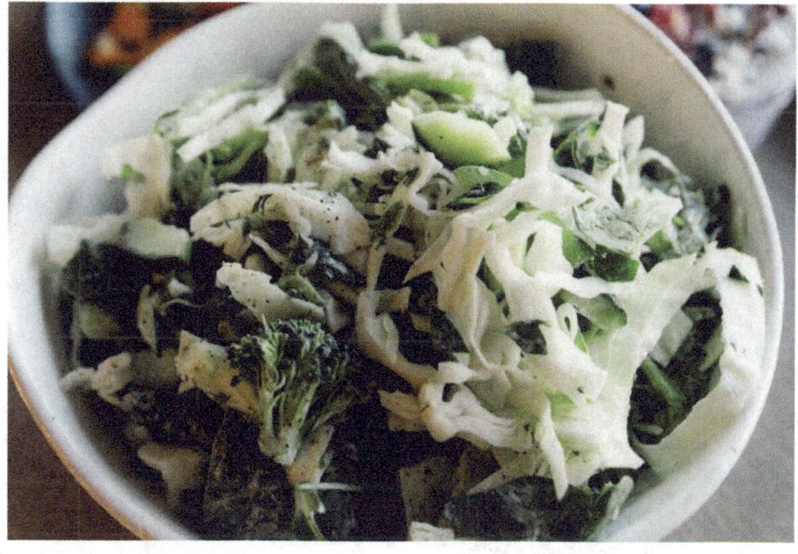

Ingredients

- 1 small cabbage
- 1 cup spinach
- 1 cup arugula
- 1 cup broccoli
- 1 large cucumber
- 1 large green pepper
- 1/4 cup green onion

Dressing

- 1/4 cup Greek yogurt
- 1 Tbsp. fresh chopped dill
- 1 Tbsp. fresh chopped cilantro
- 1 Tbsp. fresh chopped chives
- 1 Tbsp. lemon juice
- 1/4 tsp. salt

Directions

Chop cabbage, spinach, arugula, broccoli, cucumber, green pepper, and green onion into small pieces. Combine in large bowl. In a separate bowl, mix together ingredients for dressing, adding water to thin out if necessary. Drizzle over salad mix, tossing to coat full salad.

Easy Zucchini Pasta

This recipe makes 4 servings

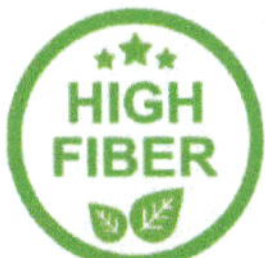

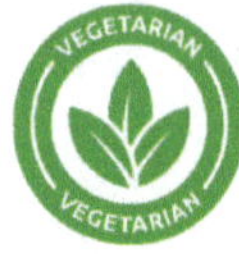

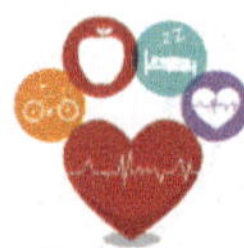

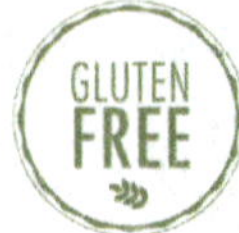

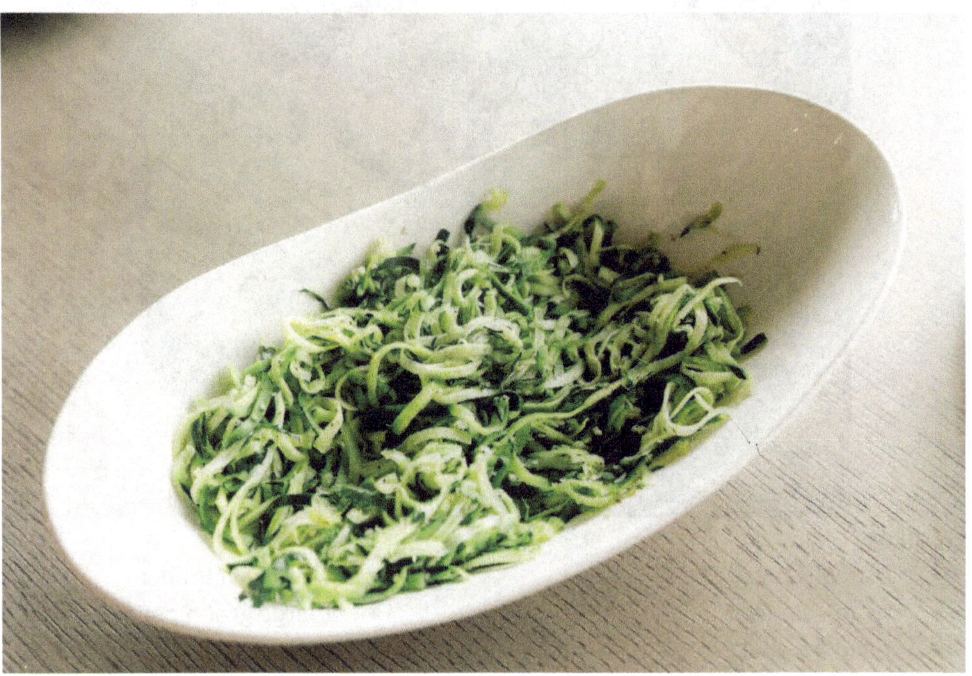

Ingredients

- 2 Tbsp. olive oil
- 1 tsp. thyme
- 3 garlic cloves, minced
- 5-6 medium zucchini, spiralized
- Parmesan, grated
- Salt and pepper to taste

Directions

In a sauté pan over medium heat, add olive oil and allow to heat. Add zucchini. garlic and thyme. Cook until tender (5-6 minutes).

CHAPTER 7: FOOD SHOPPING AND MEAL PLANNING

Now that you are beginning to learn what to eat, how can you put it into a routine? That's what this chapter is all about.

Let's save you stress, time, cash, and your waistline by planning meals! I'll break this down into four steps for you. The first step is **planning a shopping day.** The second step is **taking inventory** of all the food you have in your home. The third step is to put together a **meal plan** and a **shopping list.** And the final step is to **shop strategically**.

Plan Your Shopping Day

My first suggestion when it comes to meal planning is to pick a day that you are going to do your food shopping. I go on Sunday because I know then that the rest of the week is going to go smoothly. If I go on Sunday, I can think about what the following week looks like: Do the kids have swim meets? Am I traveling? Am I going to be working late? What do those meals look like, and how quickly do I have to prepare them? And this is also when you can think of leftovers. What are you going to have during that week?

Also, by going to the store less often, you are going to spend less money and buy what you actually need. Think about when you go to the store on random days; you might end up with something tempting that the store has purposefully displayed at the front of the store or on an endcap. You don't need those chips or cookies!

Take Inventory

What do you have on hand in your house? What do you need in your fridge, freezer, pantry, and spice rack?

Fridge

Let's begin with your fridge. Be honest with me—do you know everything that you have in your fridge? I just cleaned out my fridge the other day, and I will tell you that there were some science experiments happening in there! Mold on spaghetti sauce, in yogurt, and many cheeses! The thing is that these items were not even expired, so open those jars and containers, and make sure the food still looks (and smells) fresh.

If you are like me, you may have *somehow* ended up with multiple bottles of the same condiment. I had three bottles of ketchup—one was about a third full, one was barely touched, and one was half full. Condiments are one of those things you pick up when you are shopping *just in case* you are running low, but save yourself some money and check to see what you have in your fridge before you shop. Also, examine the chart below to see if you have anything that needs to be thrown out!

It feels pretty awesome to have a clean fridge!

So let's talk about some staples that you should always have in your fridge:

- Veggie tray (It's so convenient to have a healthy snack all prepared for you)
- Eggs (not just for breakfast—hard-boiled eggs make a great snack!) And who doesn't love "breakfast for dinner?" So easy and so nutritious!
- Plain Greek yogurt (My kids absolutely love having Greek yogurt—you can make dips out of it, use it as sour cream. You can add nuts, berries, and granola to it for breakfast. It's so versatile!)
- Bag salads (The quicker it is for you to prepare a salad, the more likely you will eat it! This is an easy way to get in one of your veggie servings every day!)

How long does food last in your fridge and freezer?

https://www.foodsafety.gov/food-safety-charts/cold-food-storage-charts

Freezer

If you happen to know what is in your fridge, how about your freezer? I frequently throw things in there and completely forget about them! Have you ever seen the Progressive commercial with the freezer analogy?

The narrator says, "Don't use your freezer as a time capsule." It's so funny because it is so true! In fact, the last time I saw the commercial, it inspired me to clean my freezer out. There were berries I picked last summer all frost bitten! What a waste! I had leftover meals that were unrecognizable! From now on, I have decided to clearly label things with dates and to look over the items at least every couple of weeks! We also invested in a vacuum sealer which will help food to last longer in the freezer.

Here are good foods to keep on hand in your **freezer**:

- Frozen fish and seafood (remember, as I said before, seafood is packed with omega-3s which are essential to consume through our foods.) I love frozen fish because it's cost effective; they're usually packaged in single fillets (super convenient if not everyone in your family likes fish; you can take out just the right amount that you need).
- Frozen fruits and vegetables (Frozen fruit is great for smoothies; they're already frozen, so you don't need ice.) And remember, frozen fruits and veggies are picked at peak season. They're so delicious, and they have a longer shelf life compared to fresh produce.
- Whole grain bread (Whenever I go food shopping, I buy two loaves of bread; I keep one in the freezer and one in the fridge; this way we never run out. One example I'll use is toast—if you have no fresh bread, just pull a slice or two from the frozen loaf and you can put it right in the toaster!)
- Ginger (I know, funny, right? But you can save ginger for up to a year in your freezer! I find that you never need the whole root for recipes. You can keep it in your freezer and pull it out to shave or mince a little off for recipes that call for it.)

Pantry:

It is so important to go through your pantry often and store any type of grain in airtight containers! Why? Grains can create a literal "flutter" of activity! One night I decided to make rice pilaf. I looked in one package of opened brown rice and there were these things moving in there—things with wings. I threw it out and decided to use wild rice—and there were the same things. Then I realized they were everywhere—in all my flours, in granola; it was crazy. I took a couple packages of these grains to the hardware store and asked the employee working at the counter what these were, and she informed me that they were pantry moths and that they are impossible to get rid of.

They are disgusting! They start out as little worms and then turn into moths. I had to throw out all my grains!

So, if you are like me and like to buy grains in bulk to save some money, make sure you put them in airtight containers! Or if you buy a package and use some of the grains, put the remainder in an airtight container. You don't want to have the nightmare of an experience that I had!

Now that I got that public service announcement off my chest, here are some items that I consider to be pantry essentials:

- Nut butters (peanut, almond, sunflower—they all have different values.) Buy one at a time; they can go rancid if you keep them too long.
- Tuna fish (This is a great go-to for lunch!)
- Whole grains (Farro is one of my favorites. You can also get brown rice or whole-grain pastas.) Remember the air-tight container rule!
- Canned items (Look for a little blue tag that says "No sodium added." If you have beans or regular canned items with salt, you can rinse many off.)
- Low sodium broths and stocks are great to have on hand. Soups and stews can be quick and easy to make.

Spices Galore!

I am a huge advocate of spices! I could write a whole book on this. And did you know that spices like turmeric and cinnamon may help to naturally increase your GLP-1 levels?[xxxix] Peek in your cupboard or spice rack. What do you have on hand? How old are they? Yes, they expire! And even if they're not expired, if they are over a year old, they lose potency. I like to write the date I purchased the spice on the top of the bottle with masking tape and after a year goes by, I toss them out.

Last time I cleaned out my spice cabinet, I had six parsley containers, a few containers of dill, and several containers of basil. Most of us don't *carefully* look in our spice cabinet before we shop; do it and you will save money and won't end up with so many containers of the same spice!

We are notorious for buying things that we already have. Be sure to go through your fridge, freezer, and pantry to see what you already have that you can use the week ahead.

Meal Planning

Earlier in this book, we talked about the Power of Five. Do you have the Power of Five when you plan out your meals for the week?

Lauren said, "My fiancé and I always evaluate our plates when we eat dinner, and we try to figure out what we can do next time to make sure we get all five food groups in portion sizes that Kelly recommends."

The following are some ways that I make meal planning easy for my family!

1.) Two of Everything
One way that I can help make sure that my family is be able to have at least four food groups at every meal is to make sure that I have the following in my cart:

- 2 different fruits
- 2 different vegetables
- 2 different proteins
- 2 different whole grains
- 2 different low-fat dairy products

You can mix and match your meals with those choices.

Some of you may object to my next recommendation when it comes to meal planning, but I promise you, it's one of the best recommendations I can give! It is also recommended by the American Heart Association recommends.

2.) Try to have fish twice a week. *Fish is high in Omega-3 fatty acids and will help fight inflammation.*

Remember when we discussed these healthy fats earlier in this book? In the Standard American Diet, we have too many Omega-6s -- especially from the vegetable oils in packaged food -- so we want to balance this out.

Fish will help create this balance big-time! This is also one of the reasons why the American Heart Association recommends eating fish twice a week.[xl]

You can purchase some frozen fish fillets like cod or salmon, or some tuna fish; try different ways to bring it in.

3.) Plan to Cook More at One Time. Having meals leftover for lunch the next day is an excellent way to keep your diet healthy!

4.) Plan out Theme Nights

For example, Monday nights can be a certain theme like Breakfast for Dinner; Tuesdays can be Taco Tuesdays; Wednesday is American night for barbecue or burgers; Thursdays can be Asian nights for your stir-fries or curry dishes. Fridays can be Fishy Fridays. You can also have a night that's for leftovers.

Themes help it become so easy to come up with four or five different meals.

Here are some other theme nights to consider:

- Meatless Mondays
- Sheet Pan Dinner Night
- Build-a-Bowl Night (Make a whole grain and then have a selection of veggies and protein choices.)
- Around the World Night (Perhaps you can try a Thai dish, a Mexican dish, an Italian dish and an African Dish? (There is such a thing as fusion! Be creative!)
- Loaded Nacho Night (Use low-fat cheese and lots of veggies.)
- Soup and Sandwich Night
- Finger Foods Fridays (There are so many healthy appetizers; offer a few choices.)
- Chili Nights in the winter (Try different varieties from the recipe section of this chapter.)
- Picnic Nights in the summer

Theme nights help you to mix things up and not get bored.

Creating a Shopping List:

When crafting your shopping list, it's vital to not only consider the foods you need, but also how they are organized in the store. Categorizing your list based on different sections of the store can be a game-changer. Start by thinking about the Power of Five to ensure you have two different items from each food group: fruits, vegetables, proteins, whole grains, and low-fat dairy products. Also, make sure you have the items you need for your meal plans.

As you organize your list, think about the layout of the store. The perimeter usually houses fresh, healthier options such as fruits, vegetables, meats, and dairy. By focusing your list on these sections, you'll naturally gravitate toward more nutritious choices. A well-organized list that matches the store layout can save you time, money, and help you make better food choices.

Shopping Strategically:

What does strategic shopping look like? When you have a plan with a list, you are going to be a smarter consumer and will also save some money in the process.

You want to shop in the perimeter of the store. In the perimeter of the store, we have our vegetables, fruits, meats, dairy, and often the frozen section. Most of the unhealthy food choices are in the middle of the store. Stick to the perimeter and you will be a healthier consumer. My patient Lauren said, "Shopping in the perimeter of the store is probably the number-one thing that has helped my fiancé and I lose weight and feel healthier. We don't buy stuff that we know is going to be bad for our bodies."

Also, never go shopping when you are hungry! If you are hungry, pick up something healthy at the store to eat before you shop. It could be a sushi roll or maybe a Greek yogurt.

If you are hungry, it's not that you'll necessarily buy more, but you may not make great choices.

Meal Prep

All right, so you just got home from the store. What do you do now? This is the time to prep. So if you bought the bulk-package of chicken, for example, take some out for the fridge and put the rest in the freezer so it doesn't go bad. Or, if you have a head of cauliflower or broccoli, cut it up. Don't be stuck being that person who has a whole lot of veggies go bad in the fridge.

I also suggest making a whole grain when you get back from the store; that way you can use it in different meals throughout the week.

Chapter 7 Summary:

- Choose a convenient day for grocery shopping based on your weekly schedule to ensure smooth meal preparation.
- Assess what you already have in your fridge, freezer, pantry, and spice rack to avoid purchasing duplicates and minimize food waste.
- Aim to incorporate a diverse range of food groups in your meals, such as fruits, vegetables, proteins, whole grains, and low-fat dairy products.
- Consider including fish in your diet twice a week for its Omega-3 fatty acids and anti-inflammatory properties.
- Make meal planning enjoyable by assigning themes to different days of the week, adding variety and preventing monotony.
- Arrange your shopping list based on the layout of the store and categorize items by food group and meal plan to streamline your shopping experience.
- Focus on the outer perimeter of the store where fresh and nutritious options like fruits, vegetables, and meats are typically located.
- Make healthier food choices and save money by refraining from shopping while hungry.
- Upon returning from shopping, prepare ingredients in advance to facilitate easier meal preparation throughout the week.
- Store perishable items correctly to prevent waste and extend their shelf life, reducing the need for frequent grocery trips.

Chapter 7 Goals:

Nutrition:

- Make sure you continue journaling what you are eating. This helps you to see if you are getting the Power of Five or at least 3-4 of those parts. Create a shopping list and plan the day you will do your grocery shopping.

Exercise:

- Walk for 30 minutes. If you walk after your meal, you will lower your blood-sugar levels and promote proper digestion.
- Stretch every morning.
- Continue doing squats.

Hydration:

- Have a glass of water when you get up.
- Have a glass between each meal.
- Have a glass at each meal.
- The total goal should be 64 ounces!

Fajita Stuffed Peppers

Serves 6 people

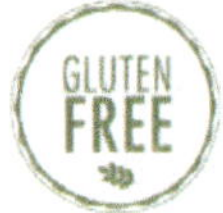

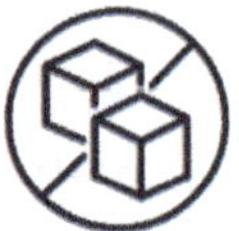
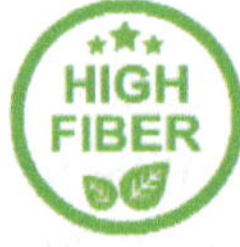

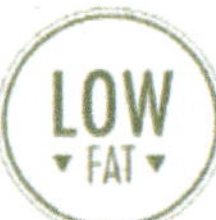

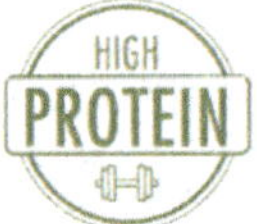

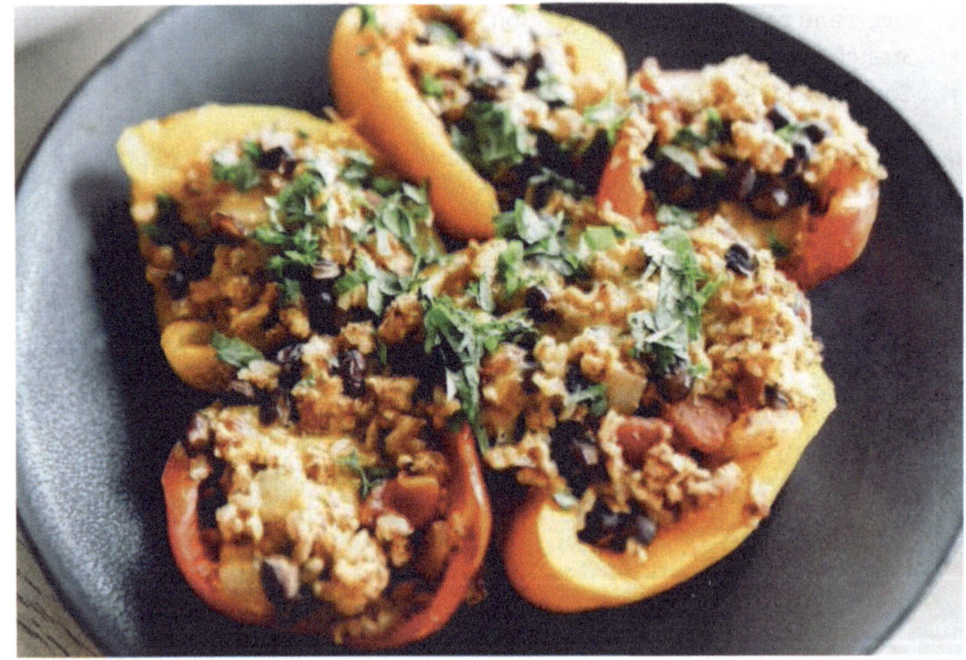

Ingredients

- 1/2 cup uncooked brown rice
- 2 tbsp. extra virgin olive oil or avocado oil
- 1 medium onion, diced
- 1 lb. 95% lean ground turkey
- 14.5 oz canned diced, no salt added tomatoes
- 15 oz. black beans, no salt added or reduced salt, drained and rinsed
- 1 tsp. chili powder
- 1 tsp. paprika
- 1 tsp. garlic powder
- 1 tsp. oregano
- 6 bell peppers
- 1/2 cup water
- 1 cup shredded, low-fat cheddar cheese

Directions

1. Preheat the oven to 400 degrees F.
2. In a small pot, prepare rice per instructions.
3. While the rice is cooking, heat up the oil in a large frying pan. Add the diced onion to the pan and cook until translucent, about 5 minutes.
4. Add the ground turkey to the pan and break up into crumbles, until turkey is fully cooked, about 10-15 minutes. Once fully cooked, drain the fat using a strainer.
5. In the pan, combine the turkey, cooked rice, diced tomatoes, black beans, and seasonings. Let the mixture simmer for about 5 minutes.
6. Add 1/2 cup of water to the bottom of the baking dish. Halve the bell peppers and remove the tops and cores. Place the 12 pepper halves onto a baking dish and distribute the rice and meat mixture evenly.
7. Sprinkle the cheese on top, and cover the dish with foil. Cook the peppers for 30 minutes; then uncover dish and cook for an additional 10 minutes.

Serve hot and enjoy!

CHAPTER 8: SNEAKY SUGAR AND SODIUM

Did you know that the average American consumes 17 teaspoons of added sugar a day, which equals about 57 pounds of added sugar a year!? Added sugar alone can lead to a host of different health problems because it causes inflammation, which can lead to type-2 diabetes, heart disease, weight gain, and many other chronic conditions we have discussed. So, we want to make sure we are monitoring how much added sugar we are consuming and where it is coming from in our diet.

We are going to talk about sodium (salt) consumption as well. Too much will raise your blood pressure, increasing your risk of heart disease and stroke. If you are like me, it may be hard to resist Chinese take-out, but did you know that a yummy sesame chicken dinner can put you over the amount of sodium you should have in a day? And then there are condiments, lunch meats, and anything packaged that surges your sodium consumption.

I know this may sound scary, telling you all the things you cannot eat, but trust me, you will not be deprived. That's unhealthy too. Remember, Kelly's Choice tagline is "Real people promoting real food." I'm more into telling you what to eat than what not to eat. Think about the plethora of one-ingredient foods on our planet; these foods do not have added sugar, and most of them have a reasonable sodium content.

I am part of the American Heart Association Board and one of my goals in advising the board members is to recommend foods for people to eat versus telling people which foods they should omit from their diet. For example, the public needs to know that reducing sodium and sugar are both beneficial for heart health.

Let's dive in and explore how sneaky sugar can be. It has even tricked me!

Natural Sugars vs Added Sugars

Once again, this comes down to looking at labels. What are we actually consuming? In January 2021, the Food and Drug Administration mandated all food companies to start including added sugars on food labels. Prior to this mandate, food companies only labeled total sugars (which included both naturally occurring and added sugars). Should we mention up here much added sugar we should be staying under each day? We could place that section "how much added sugar is okay" up here?

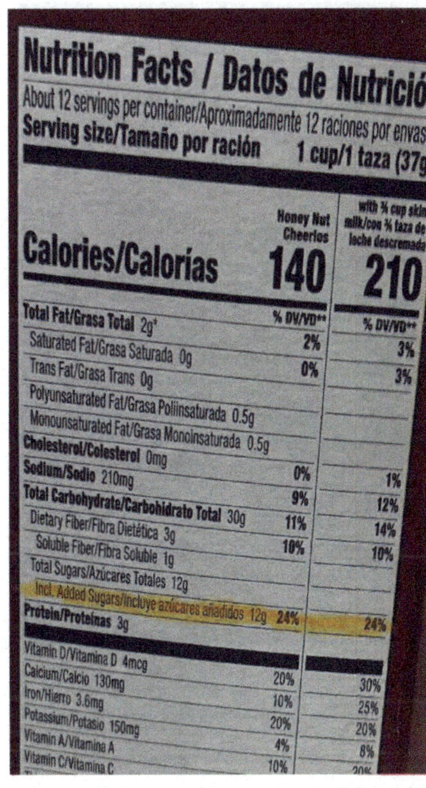

Added sugars may show up on labels as brown sugar, cane crystals, cane sugar, corn sweetener, corn syrup, corn syrup solids, crystal dextrose, evaporated cane juice, fructose sweetener, fruit juice concentrates, high-fructose corn syrup, honey, liquid fructose, malt syrup, maple syrup, molasses, raw sugar, and sugar. What about xylitol, erythritol, aspartame, etc.

The only natural forms of sugar are those that come from milk (lactose) and those that come from fruit (fructose) and honey/maple syrup. These natural sugars have added benefits like vitamins and nutrients; also, the protein in milk products and the fiber in fruit products help prevent the spike in blood-sugar levels that added sugar causes.

Added Sugar in Beverages

One of the biggest culprits of added sugar in our society is soda! Each bottle of soda has about 15-17 teaspoons of sugar. I was teaching about this at a worksite recently. To illustrate the amount of sugar in soda, I grabbed 17 teaspoons from the cafeteria and lined them up. Put that visual in your head; that is how much sugar you are consuming when you have soda (is this a visual we can actually put in the book?). That sugar is going to trigger an insulin response, which is also going to trigger your body to store that carbohydrate as fat because your body can't use it all at one time. Also, carbohydrates store as glycogen in your liver, which causes fatty liver disease. Are you surprised that fatty liver disease is not caused by fat, but is caused by sugar? These are just two reasons why added sugar is such a problem.

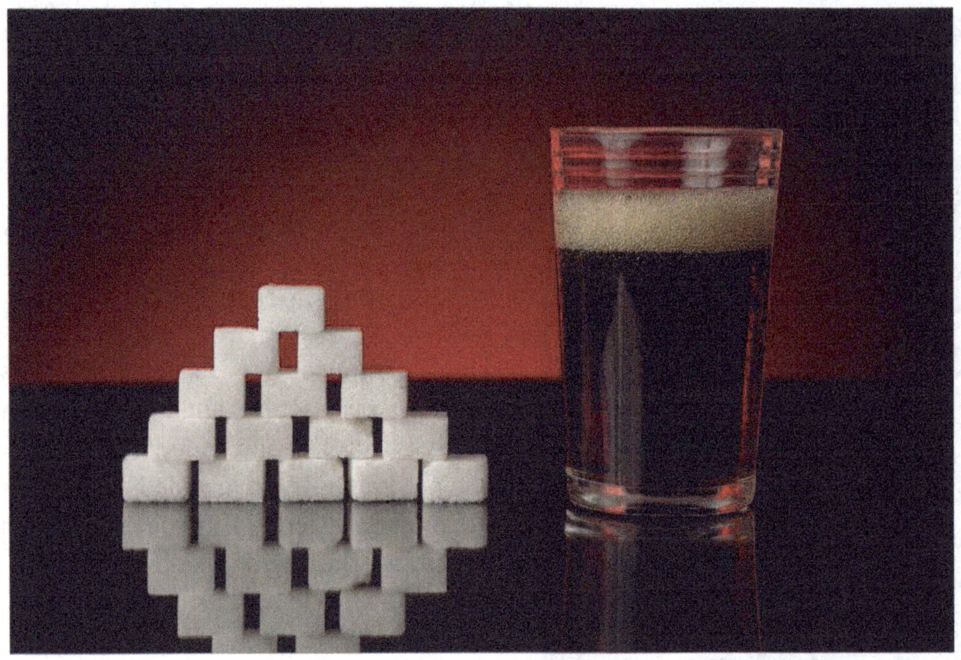

We may think about the correlation of sugar when we are talking about soda, but we may not be so quick to think about it with lemonade, iced tea, or a commercial smoothie drink. These also have tons and tons of added sugar. And those fancy coffee drinks are loaded with added sugar, too!

So be careful!

My patient Stephen was once so proud to tell me that he made a better beverage choice than soda earlier that day for his lunch. He had mango iced tea. We decided to look up the ingredients together and we were both shocked to find out that it had 137 grams of sugar! That is more than 34 teaspoons of sugar; double the amount of sugar in a typical soda.

Note that 4 grams of sugar = 1 teaspoon

As I said earlier, I can be tricked too. I can remember this one time when I had a break during a conference. I hit up a pizzeria (I did tell you I'm a pizza addict, right?). Well, didn't this restaurant have a deal; two slices and a large drink for $5? Of course, I'm going to take advantage of it even though the fountain drink choices were soda, iced green tea, and lemonade.

It was a hot day—a perfect day for iced green tea, so that's what I chose. And hey, green tea has a lot of antioxidants, so it had to be the best choice, right? It was way sweeter thanhow I make my own, but I still enjoyed it. An hour later, in the middle of a presentation on digestive health, I was nodding off. I suddenly felt exhausted. And I got called out on it—how embarrassing! My blood sugar was dipping, big-time, because of the darn iced tea!

Later that night, I had to investigate. I was flabbergasted; my iced tea had over 60 grams of sugar! That's 15 teaspoons—just as bad as soda! And sugar was the first ingredient of course, not green tea!

Other Common Foods Where Added Sugar Lurks

You can also find added sugar on a lot of foods that are down those center aisles in the grocery store. Make sure to examine your fruits in cans or jars; there can be a lot of added sugar there! When buying canned fruit, look for fruit in water or fruit juice. Canned fruit in syrup contains added sugar. A common source of added sugar in the grocery store can be protein bars, breakfast bars, cereals, and granola bars. Oftentimes, granola and protein bars are marketed as health foods. However, knowledge is power. Be a smart consumer and carefully read labels when making food choices.

My patient Tim was having three or four granola bars a day, considering them a healthy snack, until he learned that each bar had about 15 grams (which is equal to about 3 2/3 teaspoons) of added sugar.

There's another food that is misconceived as being healthy where added sugar comes into play. Even though yogurt and yogurt drinks are dairy, many food companies add a lot of sugar to these products—so read the labels!

Also watch your condiments and creamers; these are often loaded with added sugar. I'll say it again—read the labels!

How Much Added Sugar Is Okay?

Women should have no more than 6 teaspoons of added sugar a day—about 25 grams. And men should have 9 or less teaspoons—about 36 grams. So, think about that—just one flavored yogurt and a flavored coffee beverage may put you over the edge.

If you are taking GLP-1 medications, it is crucial to be mindful of your added sugar intake. In a study that was conducted to determine if there was a correlation between the consumption of dietary added sugars and the GLP-1 response, it was found that "independent of sex, adiposity, or physical activity levels, dietary added sugar consumption is associated with striatal reactivity to food cues."[xli]

When I read this study, I must admit, I had no idea what striatal reactivity to food cues meant so I had to research it. Let me break it down for you:

- **Striatum:** This is a region deep inside the brain that's involved in processing rewards, motivation, and decision-making. It's like the control center for our responses to things we find rewarding or pleasurable.
- **Reactivity:** This term refers to how sensitive or responsive something is to a stimulus. In this case, it's about how the striatum responds when it sees or senses something related to food.
- **Food cues:** These are signals or triggers that tell our brains that food is available or nearby. Food cues can be anything that reminds us of food, like the sight or smell of food, the sound of cooking, or even seeing a picture of food.

So, when scientists talk about "striatal reactivity to food cues," they're studying how active or responsive the striatum is when it encounters these signals that indicate the presence of food. This research helps us understand how our brains process information about food and how that might influence our eating behaviors and decisions.

The association between added sugars and striatal reactivity to food cues in this study suggests that consuming added sugars, especially in high amounts, may lead to overeating or unhealthy eating behaviors due to changes in brain activity and can lower the effectiveness of GLP-1 medications.

Additionally, A 2021 study[xlii] of 72 participants with obesity revealed that those with high added sugar intake experienced the smallest increase in GLP-1 levels following glucose consumption.

What About Artificial Sweeteners?

Sadly, when I started my education in dietetics, we were taught to recommend artificial sweeteners to people with type-2 diabetes and other health conditions. We don't do that anymore. The reason why is because these artificial sweeteners can affect your gut bacteria in a negative way. The latest research shows that not only do artificial sweeteners harm your gut bacteria, they also make healthy gut bacteria become pathogenic, meaning they can cause disease.[xliii] The latest research has shown that artificial sweeteners may even cause cancer.[xliv]

These are common artificial sweeteners you may encounter in food and beverages:

- Acesulfame potassium (Sweet One, Sunett).
- Advantame.
- Aspartame (NutraSweet, Equal).
- Neotame (Newtame).
- Saccharin (Sweet'N Low).
- Sucralose (Splenda).

How You Can Fulfill Cravings without Added Sugar:

First, you want to look for "low sugar" on labels.

When it comes to soda, many of my patients turn to flavored seltzer water instead.

My patient Michael said, "I have completely replaced soda with seltzer water. We make sure to have these in the house instead of soda, and that is what we have whenever we crave soda. It works!"

Plain Greek yogurt almost always has minimal sugar, and it is a great protein source as well. You can add your own fruit (which we know would be "natural" sugars) instead of the syrupy fruit you find in the bottom of most flavored yogurts. Plus using whole fruits gives you a fiber bonus! Also consider adding vanilla extract to plain yogurt. It's going to add that wonderful sweetness without the added sugar.

Make your own trail mix with raw nuts and a bit of dried fruit for a snack instead of sugary granola bars.

When it comes to alcoholic drinks, be smart there as well. Use seltzer water or club soda, not tonic or coke for mixed drinks.

Also, there are two sweeteners that are great sugar replacements: stevia and monk fruit. These have zero calories but a very high sweetness. You can buy them in little packets to add to your tea or coffee. They are so sweet that ½ a packet is sweeter than 3-4 regular sugar packets.

Honey and maple syrup, used sparingly, are also great sweeteners as they have health benefits. Use raw honey, which has propolis; this may help lower triglyceride levels and improve cholesterol. Honey has also been shown to be great for your immune system. Maple syrup is a phenomenal source of manganese, which helps with fat and carbohydrate metabolism, calcium absorption, blood sugar regulation, and brain and nerve function.

Sneaky Sodium

Now that we have gone over the added sugar that lurks in food, it is time to look at sneaky sodium. In the last chapter, we reviewed cans that say, "No sodium added." Let's dive a bit deeper into this.

Head to those center aisles in the grocery store, and you will find a lot of sodium. Sodium hangs out in processed food. Soup and frozen meals immediately come to mind.

How Much Sodium Should You Get Each Day?

The general recommendation is to have about 2,300 mg per day; that is just one teaspoon my friends! The American Heart Association limits sodium intake to 1,500 mg if you are at an increased risk for a heart attack. An example risk factor is high blood pressure.

The average American is getting about 3,400 mg of sodium per day[xlv]. Or… "is exceeding the recommended daily sodium limit." This is because sodium intake is not coming from your saltshaker. It comes from preservatives in your food.

Why Is Too Much Sodium a Bad Thing?

The main problem with sodium is that it causes water retention, which can then lead to high blood pressure, inflammation, and a host of health ailments,

High blood pressure is related to heart disease and stroke, two of the leading causes of death in the United States.

Study after study has found that sodium causes high blood pressure. And reducing sodium intake can lower your blood pressure. A 2020 meta-analysis published in the *British Medical Journal* showed that lowering sodium intake lowers blood pressure, especially for those who already have high blood pressure.[xlvi]

So, we go back to a message you have seen many times in this book: Eat real food! When you're eating real food—strawberries, chicken, fish, broccoli, etc.—you won't have to worry about those sodium levels like you do with processed foods.

Sprinkling some salt on your food is not going to hurt your health. You do need some because sodium is a natural electrolyte that gets water in and out of your cells. This is particularly important during and after high-intensity workouts. Think about your sweat—it's salty right?! You do need to replenish that! We don't want to take sodium out completely.

Eliminating salt can make you sick. My patient Terry was told by her doctor to limit her sodium intake because of her high blood pressure and kidney disease. She didn't just limit it; she eliminated it! She became so fatigued she could barely move. Some sodium is needed; your cells need water to function, and sodium is the gateway for water to get into those cells!

We just want to make sure we're not eating those processed foods with sky-high sodium levels.

By sky-high, here are some high-sodium foods to watch out for:

- Soup
- Jarred sauces
- Bread and bagels
- Frozen meals
- Jerky
- Salted nuts (raw nuts are delicious, I promise)
- Deli meats
- Pizza—bummer, I know
- Cheese
- Canned beans

- Italian seasoning dressing mix
- Sloppy Joe, taco, beef stew, chili spice mixes

Fortunately, consumer research has informed food companies that we want less sodium in our food.

Two 2014 studies by the CDC showcased what Americans believed about sodium.[xlvii] One study published in the *Journal of Child Nutrition & Management* illustrated that 90% of adults supported policies to lower sodium in school cafeteria foods. The other study, published in the *American Journal of Preventive Medicine,* found that most consumers thought it was a good idea for the government to keep excess sodium out of quick-service restaurant meals (82%) and manufactured foods (56%.) Almost half of consumers agreed it is a good idea to limit sodium in full-service restaurant meals (47.)

Food manufacturers have heard you, and more are offering low-sodium options year after year. Look for those low-sodium foods!

Take canned tomatoes for example. A typical can of tomatoes has about 340 mg of sodium per serving. A can of tomatoes with the "low sodium" label has about 5 mg of sodium. Food companies have been able to remove a lot of the sodium from food because they have learned that the heating process of the food preserves the food more so than sodium. If you have a pantry filled with canned tomatoes that do not have the low sodium label, you can rinse them to reduce the sodium content by 40 percent. This goes for any canned foods like beans or vegetables.

Here's an illustration of how one patient, Sam, changed up his typical Standard American Diet (SAD) to reduce added sugar and sodium intake.

Sam's SAD Food Choices	Sam's Real Food Choices
Breakfast:	**Breakfast:**
Sugary cereal with whole milk	Muesli with berries and skim milk
Doughnut	Peanut butter on whole-grain toast
Lunch:	**Lunch:**
Fast food roast beef sub	Chicken breast sandwich with lettuce,tomato and avocado on whole wheat roll
Canned soup with saltines	Low sodium canned soup with whole-grain Triscuit crackers
Snack:	**Snack:**
Candy bar	Ants on a log
Sugary granola bar	KIND bar
Dinner:	**Dinner:**
Taco with taco seasoning mix	Taco Stew at the end of this chapter
Chef salad with Italian seasoning mix	Butternut Squash Salad recipe at the end of this chapter

How to Reduce your Sodium Intake at Home

An easy way to reduce sodium within your diet is to cook more at home. Here are tips for adding flavor to home-cooked meals without sodium:

a. Experiment with spices like thyme, cumin, basil, oregano, and turmeric.
b. Citrus adds so much flavor! Squeeze lemon, lime, or orange on your meat and veggies!
c. Experiment with vinegars (white and red wine, rice wine, balsamic, and flavored balsamic—like raspberry).
d. Add heat with chopped fresh chili peppers or dried options like cayenne or red pepper flakes.
e. Toasted sesame seeds or walnuts can add a lot of flavor.

Chapter 8 Summary:

- The average American consumes excessive amounts of added sugar, contributing to inflammation, type-2 diabetes, heart disease, and weight gain, making it crucial to monitor added sugar intake. Added sugar may also affect the effectiveness of GLP-1 medications. Aim for staying under 25 g of added sugar per day for women...

- Acknowledging the difference between natural and added sugars is essential; natural sugars found in milk and fruits come with added benefits like vitamins and fiber, while added sugars hide in various forms on food labels and commonly in beverages like soda, lemonade, and flavored coffee drinks.

- Beverages like soda, lemonade, and iced tea can contain alarming amounts of added sugar, leading to potential health risks, with some surprising choices harboring more sugar than expected.

- Added sugars lurk in unexpected foods like canned fruits, granola bars, yogurt, and condiments, making it essential to read labels carefully and be mindful of daily intake limits.

- The association between added sugars and striatal reactivity to food cues in this study suggests that consuming added sugars, especially in high amounts, may lead to overeating or unhealthy eating behaviors. This is due to changes in brain activity and can lower the effectiveness of GLP-1 medications.

- Formerly recommended as alternatives, artificial sweeteners can negatively impact gut health and may even pose cancer risks, leading to a shift towards natural alternatives like stevia and monk fruit.

- Fulfilling cravings without added sugar involves opting for low-sugar options, like incorporating plain Greek yogurt with fresh fruits, making homemade trail mix, and using sweeteners like honey and maple syrup sparingly for health benefits.

- Excessive sodium consumption, primarily from processed foods, can lead to water retention, high blood pressure, heart disease, and stroke, emphasizing the importance of monitoring sodium intake and choosing low-sodium alternatives. 2,300 mg or less per day.

- Tips for reducing sodium intake include cooking at home more often, experimenting with herbs, spices, and citrus for flavor, and choosing low-sodium options while eating out to promote heart health and overall well-being.

Chapter 8 Goals:

Nutrition: Look at added sugar and sodium levels on all labels.

Exercise: Walk for 30 minutes; continue stretching; and try doing 10 bicep curls every day! And then do 10 sit and stands from a chair.

Hydration: Continue getting 64-ounces of water. Find a water bottle you love to inspire you!

Dessert Sweet Potato
This recipe makes two servings

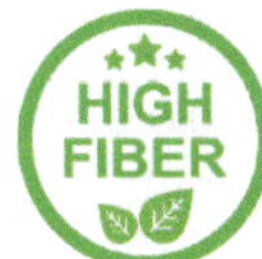

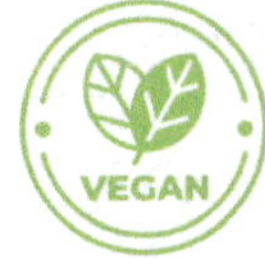

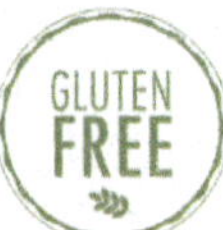

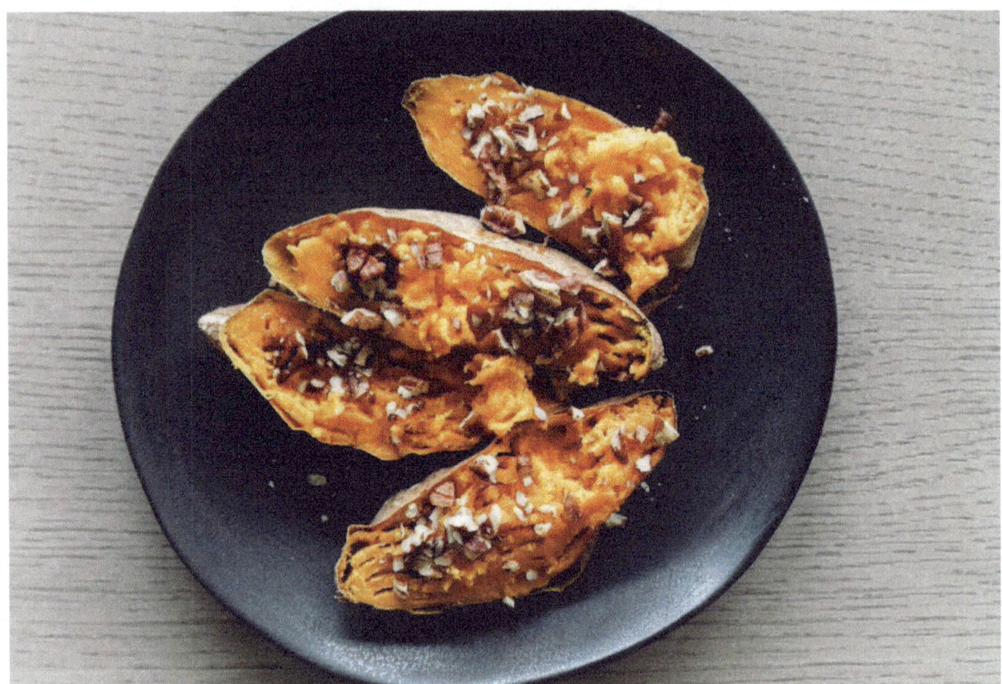

Ingredients

- 1 medium sweet potato
- 1-2 Tbsp. pure maple syrup
- 1/4 cup chopped nuts

Directions

Preheat oven to 425 degrees F. Poke holes in the sweet potato with a fork. Place the sweet potato on top of a baking sheet lined with aluminum foil or parchment paper. Bake for 45 minutes. Place sweet potato on a plate and cut open lengthwise. Top sweet potato with maple syrup and chopped nuts and enjoy!

CHAPTER 9: UPGRADING BREAKFAST AND SNACKS

We have covered the nutrients your body needs and the foods you should limit to function optimally. You have learned how to approach food shopping and meal planning. Now, we are going to train your brain to prioritize breakfast and healthy snacks.

Breakfast

Breakfast is your most important meal of the day! Do you eat breakfast every day? Research shows that 31 million Americans skip breakfast. Let's try to change that! Breakfast literally means break the fast!

If you are missing out on breakfast, you're missing out on an opportunity to consume nutrients such as fiber and protein, making it difficult to reach your daily intake goals.

The main reason individuals skip breakfast is because they are rushing out of the house in the morning! Let's face it, we are busy! Cooking oatmeal on the stove or cooking fresh eggs every morning isn't an option for everyone. Let's review some healthy options that are quick and easy! When an average American thinks about a quick breakfast, they're usually thinking about a sugary, high-carb breakfast like waffles, bagels, toast, pancakes, doughnuts or sugary cereals.

We want to make sure we're breaking the fast with something that is going to be good for our bodies. This again goes back to the Power of Five.

My first go-to is eggs. They're fantastic for you—an amazing source of protein, iodine, vitamins, minerals, and just the right amount of fat needed to absorb the vitamin D and E in the eggs. I pair this awesome protein source with a fiber source. It may be my whole grain toast or a cup of berries.

If you think you don't have time for eggs, just microwave them. Crack an egg into a mug, mix it up and maybe add some spinach or cheese in it and you have instant scrambled eggs in the microwave!

Or you can make a batch of hard-boiled eggs for the week and then you will have them ready as a grab-and-go option with fresh berries or fruit of your choice.

How to Make the Perfect Hard-Boiled Egg
Step 1: Bring your eggs to room temperature.
Step 2: Put your eggs in a pot of water before you boil them.
Step 3: Bring the water to a boil and boil them for 10 minutes.
Step 4: Pour cold water over eggs immediately after boiling them. This helps to prevent them from turning green.
Step 5: Put them in the fridge.

Another great combo is Greek yogurt with berries and ground flax or chia seeds.

There's one more breakfast idea I want to share with you: overnight oats! You can actually cook oats overnight in your refrigerator! Get a mason jar, pour in oats, add milk of your choice, and berries of your choice. Place the mason jar in your refrigerator, and the next morning it's ready to go! For exact measurements, check out the recipe at the end of this chapter.

Eating a protein and fiber-rich breakfast will boost your energy and concentration levels. It will also help prevent you from eating too much later in the day or making bad choices. Eating breakfast will also help stabilize blood sugar levels.

There are thousands of studies that have found multiple ways that eating breakfast is better for your physical and mental health.

A study conducted on middle-aged and older-aged male health professionals found that eating breakfast was associated with a lower risk of heart disease.[xlviii]

Tel Aviv University has conducted many studies about the impact of breakfast on blood sugar levels. A 2015 study[xlix] found that people with type-2 diabetes who skip breakfast have very high spikes in their blood sugar level even if they eat a lunch and dinner with good fiber and protein sources and little natural or added sugars.

The same researchers at Tel Aviv University found that adults who were obese and had type-2 diabetes lost more weight and had better blood glucose levels when breakfast was the biggest meal of their day, consisting of that powerful fiber and protein combo.[l]

In a 2019 study featured in Clinical Nutrition Experimental[li], researchers observed that consuming a high-protein breakfast, comprising of a minimum of 51 percent of the meal's calories from protein, triggered heightened production of GLP-1 among participants. Concurrently, participants reported feeling more satiated, resulting in decreased appetite. The researchers discussed the promising implications of these results for losing weight and regulating blood sugar levels.

A study by the American College of Sports Medicine, the American Dairy Association, and the American School Health Association found that eating breakfast at school can help kids be more attentive, behave better, and achieve higher test scores.[lii]

Breakfast can also help improve adults' performance at their jobs. A recent study[liii] of 2,000 Americans (1,000 who eat breakfast and 1,000 who do not eat breakfast) found that those who eat breakfast are more likely to get a promotion at work!

And get this—breakfast skipping can result in a crazy amount of negative consequences; in a 2020 study[liv] of nearly 22,000 college students throughout the world, researchers found that infrequent and/or frequent breakfast skipping was associated with inadequate fruit and vegetable intake, frequent soft drink intake, not avoiding fat and cholesterol, current binge drinking, current tobacco use, gambling, not always wearing a seatbelt, inadequate physical activity, inadequate tooth brushing, not seeing a dentist in the past year, and having been in a physical fight.

And that's not all! Infrequent and/or frequent breakfast skipping was also associated with depression, post-traumatic stress disorder, loneliness, insomnia and sleep problems, and poor academic performance.

Science agrees with me that you should eat a nutrient-dense breakfast!

The Snack Attack

Overall, I am not a big fan of snacking. It's important to have set mealtimes. You need to be mindful when you are eating; you will learn more about this in Chapter 11. Snacking (or grazing) can lead to overeating.

That said, a healthy snack is necessary when you have a long gap between meals. For example, if you have lunch at noon and then you don't have a meal again until 7:00

p.m., your dinner choice probably isn't going to be a great one because your blood sugar dropped too low! You're starving, and your body starts looking for those simple carbohydrates to raise your blood sugar. Plugging a snack in between lunch and dinner can help you stabilize your blood sugar until dinner.

But, think about the snack aisle at the grocery store; it's usually loaded with simple carbs: pretzels, popcorn, chips, cookies. These are not the type of snacks I'm talking about!

I want you to start thinking differently about snacks. Use the education you have received in all the chapters of this book. Take a walk down the snack aisles at the grocery store. You will see little to no fiber and minimal protein. You will see foods with high amounts of sodium and added sugar. You will see choices with a high amount of saturated or trans fats.

Processed snacks can send you on a blood sugar roller-coaster. The cookies, chips, or candy will spike that blood sugar, and then shortly after, your blood sugar will crash, and so will your energy.

I want you to think about snacks in the same way I asked you to think about breakfast. You want to go for the powerful protein-fiber combo using real food. This combination will fill you up, give you sustainable energy, and regulate your blood sugar and appetite. What does this look like?

- Nut butter and veggies. Who doesn't love ants on a log—celery with peanut butter and raisins?
- A handful of raw nuts with an apple
- Hummus and carrots
- A cheese stick and some berries

My patient Lisa was amazing at losing weight because she packed little bags of veggies and little bags of nuts with the days of the week on the bags so she would have a healthy snack choice at work instead of going to the vending machine.

An important factor when it comes to snacking is not to snack too late. I usually give my patients a cut-off time of 8:00 or 9:00 PM. As I talked about breakfast being the time of breaking our fast, we also need to give our digestion a chance to rest.

Hydration

You have hydration goals in every chapter. One of the reasons is because I have found with my patients that they are often dehydrated, which leads them to snack a little bit more. If you are eating balanced meals, you probably don't need more than one snack a day; so, if you're feeling hungry, it could be because you didn't have enough fluids that day.

Remember, we're trying to reach those 64 ounces, so hydrating yourself evenly throughout the day is going to curb that hunger.

Chapter 9 Summary:

- Breakfast is vital for kickstarting your day with essential nutrients and fiber, setting the tone for healthy eating habits.

- Incorporate protein and fiber-rich foods like eggs, Greek yogurt with berries, and overnight oats for a nutritious start to your day, even on busy mornings.

- Numerous studies have linked eating breakfast to better health outcomes, including reduced risk of heart disease, improved blood sugar control, and enhanced cognitive function.

- GLP-1 Response to High-Protein Breakfast: A 2019 study in Clinical Nutrition Experimental demonstrated that a high-protein breakfast increased GLP-1 production, promoting satiety and reducing appetite, which could aid in weight management and blood sugar regulation.

- Research shows that children who eat breakfast perform better academically, while adults may experience increased productivity and better job performance.

- Skipping breakfast has been associated with a range of negative outcomes, including poor dietary choices, mental health issues, and decreased academic performance.

- While snacking can help bridge the gap between meals, it's essential to choose nutrient-dense options like nut butter with veggies, raw nuts with fruit, or hummus with carrots to avoid blood sugar spikes and crashes.

- Staying hydrated throughout the day can curb unnecessary snacking by ensuring that hunger cues aren't confused with thirst signals, making it easier to maintain a balanced diet and manage weight.

Chapter 9 Goals:

Your Nutrition Goals: Try to find a snack you love that has protein and vegetables. Keep up your food journaling.

Your Exercise Goals: Keep up the movement. Walk 30 minutes a day and stretch every day. The best time to go for a walk is after a meal; it will help regulate blood sugar levels.

Then for strength, you want to continue 10 bicep curls, 10 sit-stands, and 10 squats every day.

Hydration Goals: Keep the 64 ounces going; if it gets boring, add some lemon or lime slices. It'll give you some flavor and add nutrients too!

Roasted Chickpeas

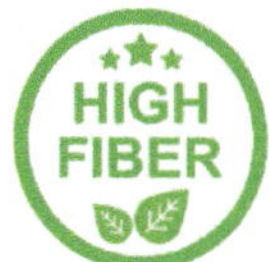

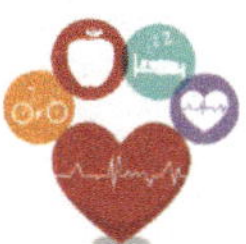
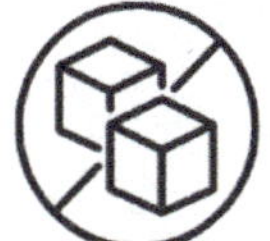
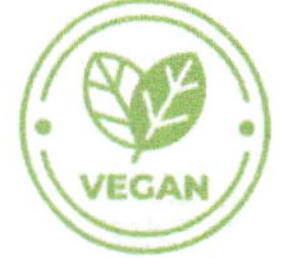

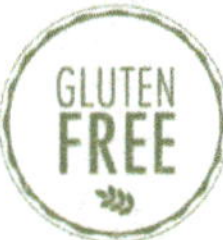

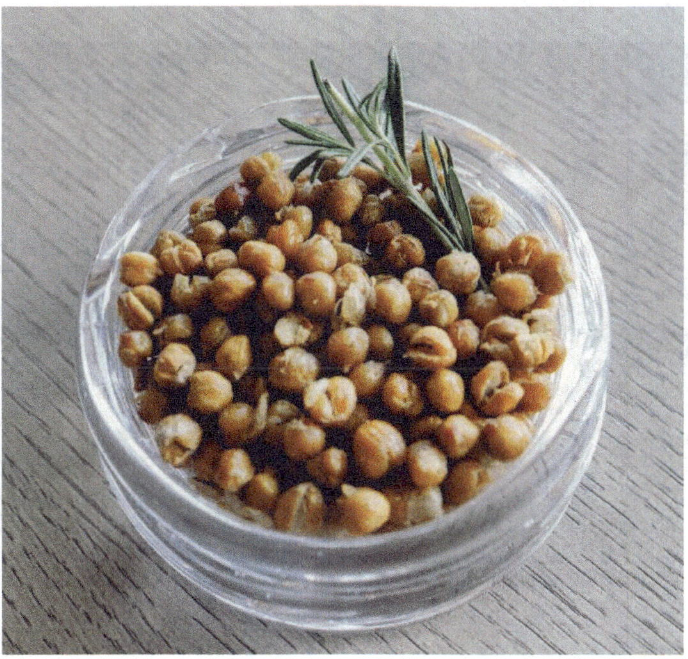

Ingredients

- One 15 oz. can of chickpeas
- Extra Virgin Olive Oil
- Sprinkle of seasoning of choice
- Sprinkle of salt

Directions

Preheat oven to 375 degrees F. Place parchment paper on a baking sheet. Pour the chickpeas into a strainer to dispose of the liquid. Pat them dry with a paper towel. Lay the chickpeas on the baking sheet and drizzle with olive oil, then sprinkle seasoning and salt. Bake in the oven for 45 minutes, shaking the pan every 10 minutes or so. Take the chickpeas out of the oven, and let them cool before eating. Enjoy!

Ham and Cheese Egg Muffins
Recipe makes 12 servings

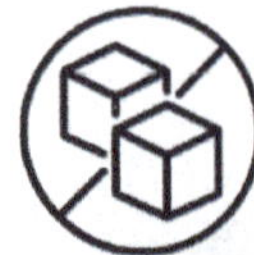
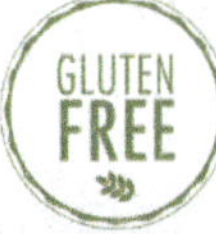

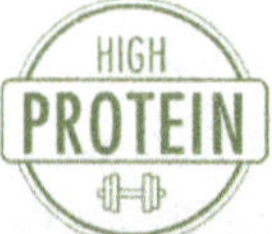

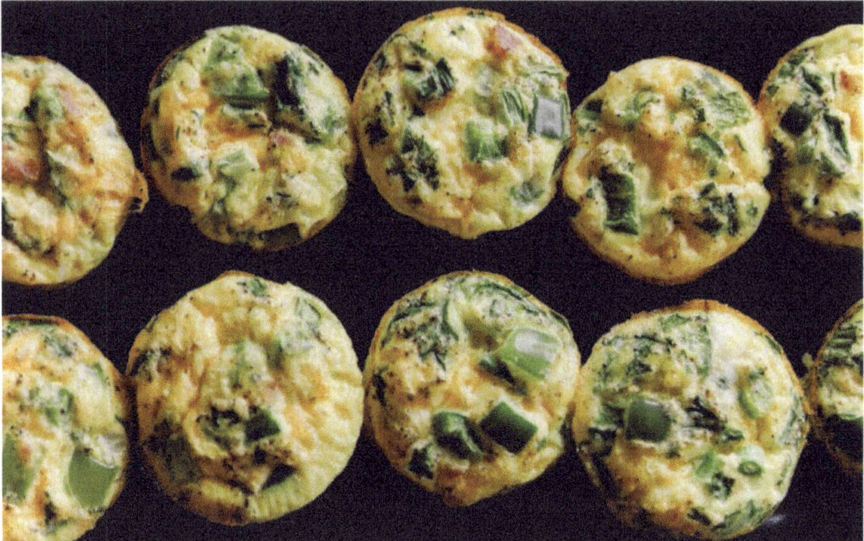

Ingredients

- 10 eggs
- 1/3 cup reduced-fat milk
- 1 cup diced ham
- 3/4 cup diced red bell pepper
- 2/3 cup reduced-fat shredded cheese
- 1/4 cup chopped green onions
- 2 Tbsp. chopped fresh parsley
- 1/4 tsp. salt
- 1/2 tsp. black pepper
- Non-stick cooking spray

Directions

Preheat oven to 375 degrees F. Crack eggs into large mixing bowl. Add milk and whisk. Add the ham, red bell peppers, cheddar cheese, green onions, parsley, salt, and pepper. Stir together. Spray a 12-cup muffin pan with non- stick cooking spray and fill q/3 of each cup with egg mixture. Bake until the eggs are just barely set, about 19-23 minutes (or until at an internal temperature of 145 degrees F). Let them cool in muffin pan for about 5 minutes.

This recipe is easy to personalize with vegetables and cheese flavor of your choice.

CHAPTER 10: SLEEP ESSENTIALS

How has your sleep been lately? Are you getting enough? Have you slept soundly through the night most nights? Maybe you have trouble falling asleep at a reasonable bedtime or falling back to sleep when you wake up in the middle of the night. If you are like most Americans, me included, your sleep is not ideal.

You should sleep 7-9 hours a night to function optimally during the day. According to the Sleep Foundation, more than 35% of American adults sleep less than 7 hours.[lv] And even if you are laying down for 7 hours, you likely are not getting a good night's sleep. This chapter is all about how you can change that and how you can assure that your sleep is restful. I will give you some nutritional and lifestyle suggestions to help improve your sleep.

How Sleep Deprivation Affects your Health

Sleep is like a battery pack. You recharge your cellphone every night; well, you need to do the same for your body. If your body is not recharged, you are looking to find energy in any form—and a lot of times, you will reach for something sugary. Simple carbohydrates will give you that quick energy boost, but that blood sugar will drop, and you will keep craving sugar throughout the day. It's not you—it's your lack of sleep. A recent study by Columbia University researchers[lvi] found that poor sleep resulted in not only lower fiber intake (sugary treats almost always lack fiber), but also, more saturated fat intake. And that's bad news for your waistline and your overall health!

Additionally, research shows that sleep disturbances (obstructive sleep apnea, insufficient or poor sleep quality have been shown to adversely affect your GLP-1 levels.[lvii]

Steps to Improving your Sleep.

- **Set a Bedtime for Yourself**

Many of you set alarms so you know when you need to wake up to be ready for your next day. Make sure you give yourself a bedtime (just like you had as a kid) to assure that you get at least those 7-9 hours of sleep. I recommend getting to bed at least 8 hours before the alarm in case you don't fall asleep right away.

- **Eject Electrical Devices from Your Nighttime Routine**

You may not like what I'm about to say, but it's important. Time for some tough love! You've no doubt heard this from other experts; you need to put away your devices and turn off the TV a few hours before bed. The blue light has been scientifically proven to reduce your body's natural production of melatonin (a hormone that helps stimulate sleep), which messes up your circadian rhythm. Technology also stimulates your mind, making it difficult to fall asleep.[lviii]

Most people I know unwind at night by watching "their show" or scrolling through Instagram. Try to do something different. Go for a stroll. Do some stretching.

My patient Denise has switched her TV habit with doing a light yoga routine before bed and her sleep has improved tremendously!

- **Say No to Sugar or Alcohol Before Bed**

I know, I know, it seems like I am restricting the good stuff, but I am simply suggesting saying no before bed! High-sugar foods like cookies, candy, or ice cream will disturb your sleep big-time. In fact, a 2016 study found that those who ate sugary snacks before bed had far less restorative sleep than those who did not eat sugary snacks before bed.[lix]

My patient Mary used to drink wine before bed because it made her sleepy. She may have fallen asleep sooner, but she was not getting enough deep sleep. She would wake up still tired! When we switched her routine from wine to herbal tea, she reported having a good night's sleep and waking up refreshed!

Caffeine can also negatively impact your sleep—so be sure you steer clear of caffeine after 2:00 p.m. The reason why is related to what is called the caffeine half-life. This means that half of the caffeine you consume is still in your system up to six hours after consumption, keeping you alert...not the most helpful state right before bedtime!

- **Journaling or Reading Before Bed**

I am a big advocate of either journaling or reading before bed. Journaling can be especially helpful at de-stressing. In a recent study[lx] of 41 college students plagued by stress, a random group of the students were assigned with the task of journaling 15 minutes before they go to bed about something positive they have experienced. This exercise improved the students' sleep time and quality.

Journaling doesn't necessarily have to be written expressions. You can simply write out your to-do list for the next day to get those tasks out of your mind and onto paper. In fact, one study[lxi] suggested that doing so can help you fall asleep more quickly.

- **Try Some Tryptophan**

Okay, so we talked about avoiding sugary foods and alcohol before bed, and now I will tell you some foods that are beneficial for sleep. Think back to your last Thanksgiving; sure you may have eaten a lot more than usual, which can make you sleepy, but, the tryptophan from the turkey can make it even more likely that you will feel sleepy. All animal products contain tryptophan because it is an amino acid. As mentioned in the protein chapter, tryptophan can help promote serotonin and melatonin, which both can help you sleep better. So, getting in some good protein throughout the day will benefit you when it comes time to go to bed.

- **Reach for Fiber-Rich Food Choices**

There's that f word again—fiber! Did you know that most of your serotonin is produced in your gut? The gut bacteria that produces serotonin can only live on fiber-rich food choices, so getting enough fiber throughout your day will help produce serotonin, which will in turn help with sleep. We'll be talking about this more in the gut health chapter.

- **Daily Movement**

Of course, movement throughout the day is going to help you have a better night's sleep. You don't need to be a marathon runner, just make sure that you get in some movement, like the exercise goals I have at the end of each chapter.

- **Make Your Bedroom Your Sleep Sanctuary**

I encourage you all to create a sanctuary for your bedroom. Do you have piles of paperwork or laundry around your bedroom? If so, you are exhibiting a form of hoarding. No judgment! Everyone gets behind on chores and organization . But it is especially important to keep the bedroom picked up. Think clean and simple. It's been scientifically proven that clutter can disrupt your sleep; a 2015 study by researchers at St. Lawrence University[lxii] found that people at risk of hoarding had poor sleep and sleep disturbances.

- **Helpful Tools**

I highly encourage blackout shades so any outdoor light or an early rising sun doesn't wake you. If you are unable to get blackout shades, try a sleep mask.

To prevent noises from disrupting your sleep, white noise machines can help. I use a fan in my room to help block out my giggling teenagers who stay up much later than my husband and I.

If you have a snoring bedmate, I recommend that you wear earplugs. But that's not all. Anyone who snores should see their family doctor for a sleep study referral. Snoring is often associated with sleep apnea. And a sleep study can be used to diagnose sleep apnea. Sleep apnea is literally pausing in breathing, which can lead to loud snoring.

You should also ask your bedmate if you snore. A bedmate will recognize this more than you will. If you do snore, then you too should see about having a sleep study!

Sleep studies are often conducted overnight in a laboratory; some doctors can conduct them by having you use a portable, take-home testing kit.

People with sleep apnea often feel fatigued throughout the day because they are not getting sufficient REM sleep, and aside from having difficulty concentrating, sleep apnea will lead to health problems the same way it does for anyone getting less than seven hours of sleep...even if the person with sleep apnea is in bed for nine hours!

Several studies have shown that having sleep apnea increases your risk of type-2 diabetes, cardiovascular disease, strokes, heart attacks, and even a shortened life span.[lxiii]

So, what can be done if you or your bedmate does have sleep apnea? Your doctor may order you a continuous positive airway pressure (CPAP) machine. You wear hoses on your nose attached to this machine when you sleep; humidified air pipes through your nose, which creates air pressure to keep your throat open while asleep; this prevents pauses in breathing.

There are more and more treatments becoming available for sleep apnea as well—even an implant that can help patients breathe better while sleeping.

Chapter 9 Summary:

- Aim for 7-9 hours of restful sleep each night to support overall health and well-being, as insufficient sleep can lead to negatively impact your health.
- Poor sleep can disrupt dietary patterns. You might then eat more fatty foods, and adversely affect GLP-1 levels, contributing to metabolic dysregulation.
- Set a consistent bedtime to ensure adequate sleep, allowing for relaxation and preparation for restorative rest.
- Put away your electronics well before bedtime so that blue light does not interfere with your sleep.
- Minimize consumption of sugary snacks, alcohol, and caffeine before bed, as they can interfere with sleep patterns and contribute to restlessness.
- Incorporate calming activities like journaling or reading to unwind before bedtime, promoting relaxation and improved sleep onset.
- Consume foods rich in tryptophan and fiber throughout the day to support serotonin and melatonin production, facilitating better sleep quality.
- Engage in regular exercise to promote overall health and enhance sleep quality, but avoid vigorous activity close to bedtime to prevent stimulation.
- Optimize your bedroom environment with blackout shades, white noise machines, and decluttering to promote restful sleep and minimize disturbances.
- If experiencing sleep disturbances like snoring or daytime fatigue, consider consulting a healthcare professional for a sleep study.

Chapter 9 Goals:

Nutrition: In your food journal, add a healthy bed-time snack. Some ideas might include a warm glass of milk, a rolled-up slice of turkey, or a handful of nuts.

Exercise: Invite a friend to exercise with you! Maybe you can ask a friend to join you in walking 30 minutes a day and then end it with 10 bicep curls, 10 sit-stands, and 10 squats. After that, you can do some stretching. I know that if I have someone waiting for me at the gym or the running trail, I am more likely to do it.

Hydration:

Keep trying to get in 64 ounces of water. Supplement that with hydrating vegetables like cucumbers, tomatoes, lettuces, or peppers throughout the day.

Turkey Spinach Quinoa Bowl
This recipe makes 2 servings

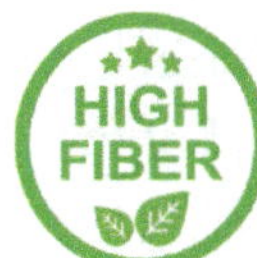

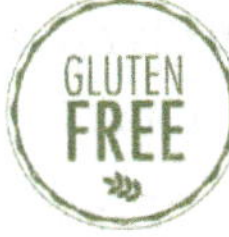

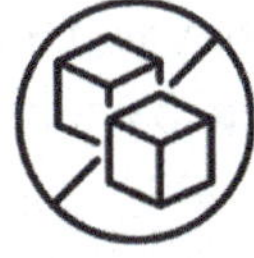
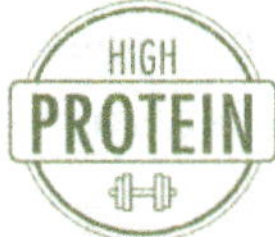

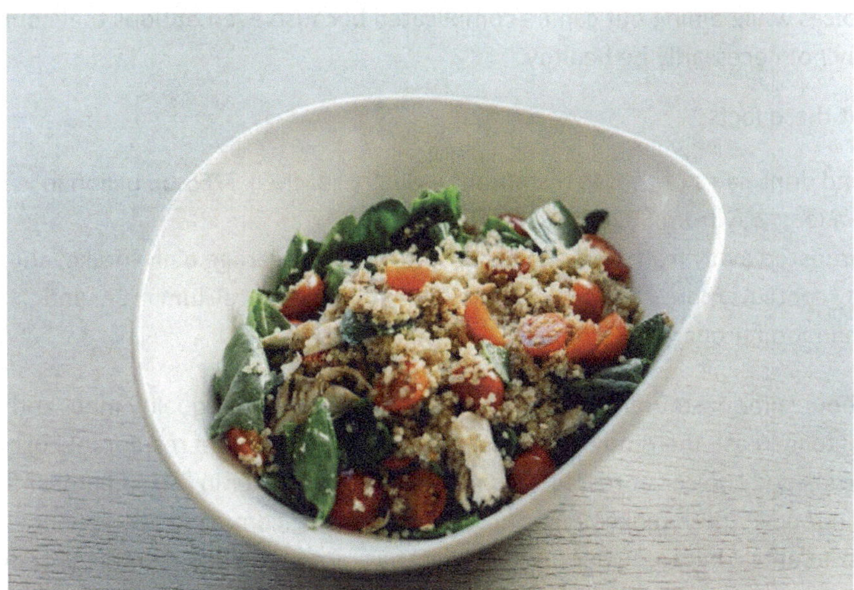

Ingredients

- 1 cup cooked quinoa
- 4 oz. cooked turkey breast, shredded
- 1 cup fresh spinach
- 1/2 cup cherry tomatoes, halved
- 1/4 cup feta cheese, crumbled
- 1 Tbsp. olive oil
- Balsamic vinegar to taste
- Salt and pepper to taste

Directions

Combine quinoa, turkey, spinach, cherry tomatoes, and feta cheese in a bowl. Drizzle with olive oil and balsamic vinegar. Season with salt and pepper. Toss gently and serve.

CHAPTER 11: DINING OUT HEALTHFULLY

This is one of my favorite chapters. To be honest with you, cooking is not my forte, but I am great at reservations. Going out to eat is a favorite pastime not just for me, but for most Americans.

Making choices while dining out can be complicated because even options that sound healthy may not necessarily be healthy.

Think about these facts:

- Food and drink sales of the US restaurant industry reached $765.06 billion in 2019—a long way from $370.5 billion seen in 1992.[lxiv]
- Food prepared away from home takes up 34% of total average daily intake, and typically contains more saturated fat and sodium, and less calcium, iron, and fiber than food prepared at home.[lxv]

Let's talk about some restaurant "tricks." One is that they buy low-quality meat and soak it in oil to increase the tenderness. Plus, the amount of sodium restaurants use is off the charts! Food choices at restaurants are going to be higher in fat, sodium, and calories than food you can make at home. Go to calorieking.com and look up your favorite restaurants. I bet that your favorite meal has more than 1,200 grams of sodium; that's more than you need in a whole day!

So, it's no surprise that dining out too often can increase your risk for developing chronic diseases (heart disease, type-2 diabetes, cancer, etc.) and decrease your lifespan.[lxvi]

This doesn't mean you should never eat out; there are ways to do so healthfully and that's what this chapter is all about. Plus, keep in mind, dining out and socializing with family and friends is ultra-important for your health!

Eating Out Healthfully

So, how *can* you eat healthfully at restaurants? I am excited to share with you some ideas. A lot of these ideas relate back to what you have already learned in this book.

Idea 1: Remember the Power of Five Concept

HEALTHY EATING TIPS
50% fruits and vegetables
50%
25% fiber-Rich carbohydrates
25%
25% protein-rich foods
25%

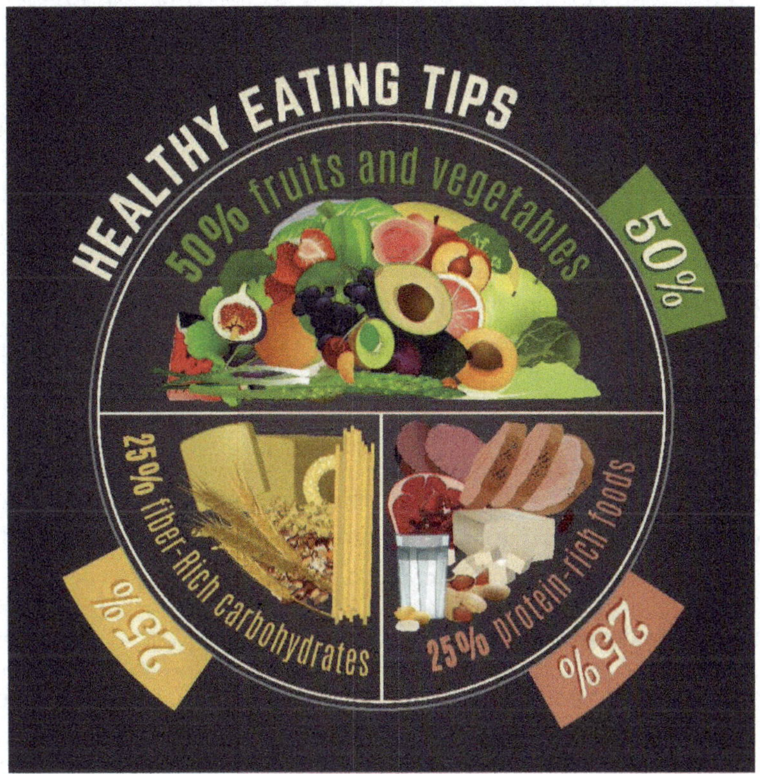

Similar to the Power of Five, for dinner at restaurants I like to include four categories—cooked veggies, raw veggies, protein, and a complex carb (whole grain). Remember, these choices help to balance calories and show you the importance of portion sizes (notice in the picture above that veggies take up *half* the plate). For instance, you wouldn't want to order an entire plate of pasta because you would only get the grain section. So, if you are craving pasta, what should you do? Order a side of pasta with some vegetables, a salad and maybe some meatballs.

I'll be frank with you—if you can make sure that half your plate is vegetables, it doesn't matter what's on the other half because those veggies are going to make sure you get fiber, cut down on the meal's calories, and give you some nutrient-dense food.

GLP-1 medications work in part by slowing down gastric emptying and increasing feelings of fullness, which can help regulate blood sugar levels and promote weight loss.

Vegetables are rich in dietary fiber, which further supports these effects by slowing down digestion, improving insulin sensitivity, and promoting satiety. By ensuring that half of your plate is filled with vegetables, you will increase your fiber intake, which may enhance the efficacy of GLP-1 medications in managing blood sugar levels.

Also, the nutrient density of the vegetables will help prevent the nutrient deficiencies that GLP-1 medications can cause.

Look at the menu and see if they have grilled veggies, salad, etc. You can take options from different meals and combine them together. You don't want to drive your server crazy, but you can do this! Every time I am out to eat, people always ask me what I got because it looks amazing. That's because I combine options from different meals.

Sometimes restaurants even have leaner, healthier choices on their menu that lists the calories.

So, go for a half plate of veggies, a lean protein source, and a tiny bit of carbohydrates because you know that bread is going to be served. And if you are like me, I like a glass of wine with my dinners—so the carbs can add up quickly!

Idea 2: Leftovers Are Okay

I live walking distance to about seven different restaurants, so I have become familiar with the portion sizes at each restaurant. One of these restaurants is an Italian restaurant, and the portion sizes are huge! I know this fact beforehand, so I plan for leftovers for lunch the next day.

If you try a new restaurant that you have never been to, I want you to look mindfully at the plate. Portion sizes have grown tremendously over the years. In fact, a recent study found that serving sizes in restaurants increased by 226% between 1986 and 2016.[lxvii] And research shows that people will inevitably eat more when given larger portions.[lxviii]

A lot of times, meals are served on platters, not plates! So, assess your plate and determine what you will eat there and what you can bring home for leftovers.

Remember, knowledge is power; you know that the portion they give you will be too large! So, plan accordingly!

Idea 3: What to Avoid on a Menu

There are ways that food is prepared that increases the fat content and the calories, so if you avoid those foods, you will likely have a healthier meal. Here are some red-flag terms:

- Au gratin
- Fried (other terms for fried are battered, crispy, crunchy)
- Creamy
- Glazed
- Pan-fried
- Cheesy
- Loaded
- Fritter
- Buttery
- Bisque

A lot of times, you need to read the description of the menu item to know what you are actually getting. For example, my husband and I were out to eat at a restaurant recently and he wanted to order the Utica Greens. This is an Upstate-NY thing, and it sounds healthy, right? Well, it was probably the unhealthiest thing on the menu!

One of my friends is a doctor; and he didn't know that Utica Greens are basically greens smothered in mayonnaise with bacon and cheese until he read the description!

I hope you don't think I'm depriving you of yummy foods; there are dozens of delicious options that are prepared healthier. Steamed, broiled, baked, and grilled options are healthier. A lot of times you can even ask for something on the menu that is fried to be broiled or grilled instead.

My patient Mike said, "I always ordered fried fish until I learned not to after my Dining Out lesson from Kelly. I started ordering my fish broiled, and I was so surprised—I actually liked it better than fried fish!"

Idea 4: Eat Slowly

Enjoy conversations with friends, and eat slowly. I have a hard time with this myself! Here's a fun tip that I have tried, and it works wonderfully; put down your fork and knife between bites and it will slow you down! Drinking water will help with this too. Remember, hydration is crucial anyway!

Also, if you eat fast, your brain won't have time to tell you that you are full until after the fact!

Idea 5: Sharing is Caring

If you have trouble finding lighter options, share these meals. As I mentioned before, portion sizes tend to be large when dining out; by sharing meals, you will be cutting down on calories. Some restaurants even have half-plate options; I love this option because you can still taste delicious food, but you are not getting all the calories.

Idea 6: Look Up the Menu Before You Go Out to Eat

It can be fun to look up a menu before you go out to eat and have a plan to help you choose something that is delicious and healthy.

Idea 7: Use calorieking.com or myplate.gov to Look Up Meals

These are both great resources for chain restaurants that will show you the calories, sodium content, added sugars, grams of fat, etc. to help you make a meal choice before you even get to the restaurant.

Idea 10: Be the First to Order

When you order first, you are not going to be swayed by another person's choices.

Idea 11: Try New Proteins

Maybe you always order chicken when you dine out; try seafood instead. Also, check out the vegetarian options; these are becoming more popular, and I have had some delicious vegetarian and even vegan meals at restaurants.

Chapter 11 Summary

- Dining out is a popular activity for many Americans, contributing significantly to food and drink sales in the restaurant industry, which reached $765.06 billion in 2019.
- Choices made while dining out can be complex, as even seemingly healthy options may not always align with health goals.
- Restaurants employ various tactics, such as using low-quality meat soaked in oil and excessive sodium, which can contribute to higher fat, sodium, and calorie content in meals.
- Regularly dining out has been associated with an increased risk of chronic diseases like heart disease, type-2 diabetes, and cancer, emphasizing the importance of making healthful choices when eating out.
- A balanced approach to dining out involves mindful choices and strategies to support health goals while enjoying restaurant meals.
- Implementing the "Power of Five" concept, where half the plate comprises vegetables, along with lean protein, whole grains, and limited carbohydrates, can help create balanced and nutritious meals.
- For individuals taking GLP-1 medications, prioritizing vegetable consumption can enhance the medication's effects by increasing fiber intake and supporting nutrient density.
- Strategies such as planning for leftovers, avoiding certain menu items like fried or creamy dishes, and choosing lighter preparation methods like grilling or broiling can promote healthier dining-out experiences.
- Additional tips include eating slowly, sharing meals, reviewing menus beforehand, utilizing online resources for nutrition information, being the first to order, and experimenting with new proteins and vegetarian options to diversify dining experiences.
- Prioritizing vegetable consumption helps prevent nutrient deficiencies often caused by GLP-1 medications, and ensures adequate intake of essential vitamins and minerals for overall health.

Chapter 11 Goals:

Nutrition:Try *to* use at least one of the tips I mention in this chapter when eating out.

Fitness: You can continue to do the series of exercises I recommended in the last chapter, or you c an go to YouTube and find an exercise video to try out! Look for full-body weight, yoga, at-home Pilates, or kettle bell workouts, for some ideas.

Hydration: Keep up the 64 ounces, and I want you to try a challenge as well—at a restaurant, swap out the appetizer with a seltzer or water.

CHAPTER 12: EATING MINDFULLY

Mindfulness is getting a lot of attention lately—particularly in terms of reducing stress, but what does it mean to eat mindfully? Mindful eating is eating slowly without distractions. It's completely tuning in to what you are eating and how it makes you feel.

Eating mindfully has so many health implications. For instance, if you are tuned out of a meal, you can decrease your digestive ability by 30-40 percent! But if you are like me, you may find that eating mindfully is difficult. We are in a culture of multitasking and doing so many things at once.

The last time I realized that I was not eating mindfully was when I was driving to a presentation, eating a sushi roll, and trying to schedule a patient on the phone. I went to reach for another piece of sushi roll and realized I had eaten the entire thing with no memory of it. Multitasking while driving is very dangerous, so I don't recommend it; however, I thought this was the perfect example of how we are programmed to do so many things at once because of our go-go-go culture.

It is hard to deprogram these patterns and develop mindful practices, but once you practice this, it is going to help you with your waistline and your health.

In this chapter, we will discuss four steps to mindful eating—arriving at the food, awakening, tuning into the body, and the service around the food.

Arriving at the Food

Let's dive into the first step—arriving at the food. You may be thinking, "What in the world does that mean?" This was my patient Dave's reaction when we started this part of his transformation program. He said to me, "Kelly, I open the cupboards or fridge, pull out what I am going to eat, and eat it. How else would I *arrive* at my food?"

What I mean by arriving at the food is that you bring food into your space. Whether you are being served at a restaurant or are making a plate for yourself, those are all foods arriving in your space. Even grabbing a handful of nuts or candy would count as arriving at the food. Whatever food is coming into your space, I want you to take 30 seconds to assess it... What color is it? What I find when I work with college students for example, is that all the food is brown—potato chips, French fries, cereal; etc. So, think about that for minute—is there a variety of color on your plate?

Is half your plate veggies? Do you know what ingredients make up the meal you are eating? Is this food a Frankenfood, which means the food is all chemicals? Just taking that 30 seconds to assess what you are about to eat may help you to think about that food a little bit better. Do you need to add more vegetables? Do you have enough protein? What about fiber? Is there too much or too little food on your plate? Will the food satisfy you? How will you feel after eating the food?

Awakening

The next step is Awakening. This is when you take the first bite of your food—actually tasting your food (what a novel concept!) For me, it really is. I have three older brothers, and I was programmed from a very early age to eat as fast as possible to make sure I got my portion. And then through school, even faster. And then as a mom, it became supersonic speed. So, I am programmed to rush through eating, and I swear that there are a ton of times that I never even taste my food.

I have learned to sloooowww down. If you are taking GLP-1, it is especially important for you to slow down and arrive at your food. If you overeat, you will feel very sick to your stomach afterwards.

When we eat, we need to pause and think about the flavors, what it tastes like, and incorporate all your senses...What's the texture like? What's the aroma? Does your food have a sweet, savory, salty, sour, or bitter flavor, or does it incorporate all of these flavors?

When I took my first mindful eating course at Syracuse University years ago, we did this experiment that has stuck with me ever since. This experiment was done using a saltine. They had us take a bite out of a saltine cracker and hold it in our mouths for just fifteen seconds. And in that amount of time, the bite turned from salty to sweet. The amylase, an enzyme in your saliva, breaks down that saltine, and makes it taste sweet. It's so interesting, I had never eaten a saltine so slowly to realize this taste change.

So, when we are coming into our food and tasting our food, we enjoy it so much more. This is where you can put down the fork and the knife in between bites, and savor your food. The other thing that you are going to be able to experience by actually tasting your food is the variety of flavors.

The first time I was *awoken*, I guess you could say, was shortly after a class. I was in California and had this amazing sushi roll. The reason why this stuck with me is because I could taste all these "new" flavors in my sushi roll. It was sweet from the barbecue sauce, salty from the soy sauce, and had a savory flavor from the seaweed.

By eating slowly, I was able to enjoy all those flavor profiles.

Tuning into Your Body

After Awakening , it's time to Tune into Your Body. This is where you need to slow down, so your brain can catch up with your stomach.

When I worked in bariatrics, we taught our patients to chew each bite thirty times! Now that's excessive, but it's because we needed the food to pass through slowly. After the first day working with patients on chewing, I went home that night, and we happened to have pizza for dinner. I took a bite about the size of my head, chewed it three times, and swallowed. I realized that I do not chew my food; I inhale it like a Hoover vacuum.

So, this is where I truly had to practice this and still do—chewing quickly is a hard habit to break! So, I am going to task you with the goal to chew 10-15 times per bite. By doing this, you are going to tune into the body. You are going to be aware of what you are eating and will realize when you are full.

By putting down the fork and the knife, this is going to help you with the chewing. I know that if I don't put down my fork, I already have it fully loaded after one bite of the food in my mouth.

So, put down the sandwich; put down the fork and knife in between bites, and I can guarantee you that the challenge I am proposing will be so much easier to accomplish.

There have been a lot of studies on mindful eating. One of the coolest studies on this topic I ever found was conducted by researchers at Cornell University on two groups of people. One group was given a bowl of soup and were asked to describe their fullness after consuming it. For the most part, they were very satisfied. Another group was also given soup, but they did not know that soup was being filled from the bottom of the bowl. They just kept eating.[lxix] This shows the importance of tuning into the body; when are you actually full? Are you part of the clean plate club? Don't use yourself as a human trash can. When you are full, stop!

Think about watching a baby or a toddler eat. They cry when they're hungry, and then they push their food away or throw it when they are full. They are able to understand when they are hungry and when they are full. They listen to their bodies!

We eat so much food, and there is so much food in our spaces all the time; and for many of us, food is so abundant everywhere that we sometimes lose track of when we are hungry or full. Try to start getting cues from your own body when you are hungry and full. Ask yourself questions—What am I eating? What am I tasting? Is this food satisfying?

For individuals relying on GLP-1 medication, attuning to your body's signals becomes paramount. By cultivating this awareness, you can foster intuitive eating habits, making choices that are not only tasty, but also address your specific physiological requirements, such as weight loss and blood sugar regulation. Additionally, tuning into the body's cues can act as a barrier against stress-eating, a common pitfall for many. By recognizing hunger and satiety cues, you can distinguish between genuine physiological needs and emotional impulses, leading to healthier eating behaviors and improved outcomes in managing your condition. This step of mindful eating will help you tremendously when you are able to transition off the medication.

Service Around the Food

There is one more step to mindful eating that is critical for me to address, and this step has several sub-steps. This is an overall philosophy of mindful eating—it's about adding structure to your meals, and making them enjoyable and not distracted or rushed; I call this Service Around the Food.

Step 1: Sit Down.

If you have visited other countries, you'll notice that people almost always sit down to eat. Here in America, we are eating in our cars, eating standing up at our counter, always on the run! We are tuned out of the eating process. Sitting down to eat helps cue your body that it is "mealtime"—time to focus on your food.

Step 2: Put Away Your Devices and Turn Off the TV.

Again, it's about being in the moment while eating your food.

My patient John used to eat his dinner in front of the TV watching the evening news. He would always get two or three helpings of his meal, and would end up feeling bloated and uncomfortable every night. He began sitting down at the dinner table with his family most nights a week, which resulted in him feeling satisfied after one helping of dinner. I honestly think this is the biggest contributor to his impressive 30 lb. weight loss in three months.

Sitting while eating is going to aid in your digestion process and lead to a healthier, happier life.

Hundreds of research studies have drawn the same conclusion: that putting away electronic devices and avoiding eating in front of the TV have positive health implications. A 2014 study published in the per-reviewed journal, *Eating Behavior,*[lxx] found that watching television was associated with binge eating for adults who were attempting to lose weight. A 2017 meta-analysis[lxxi] of many studies found that eating in front of screens as a young adult increased the risk of obesity in adulthood.

Step 3: Make Your Table Look Beautiful.

It's as simple as using pretty plates, having a placemat, and even lighting candles. I know it may seem simple and maybe even silly, but by doing this, you are going to be tuned into the meal.

Think about the last time you ate at a fine dining restaurant: the lights were dim; the table looked beautiful. You are more likely to go slowly and enjoy the food. You can do the same thing at home. It's so easy to light a few candles; it's just about being mindful and doing that task.

After her first mindful eating session with me, my patient Lauren and her fiancé decided to buy a beautiful set of dinnerware and handwoven placemats; she also pulled out her favorite unscented pillar candles for their dinner table. She reported back to me that she could not believe how such a simple change made both of them appreciate their meals more and helped them both to be mindful of their eating. Lauren said, "It's like the setting was telling us, 'Hey you are eating dinner now. Focus on your meal and enjoy it!'"

Step 4: Try to Make Your Meals Last a Little Longer.

Try to make your meals last at least 20 minutes. This will be a way of telling you that you did it! You ate mindfully!

Step 5: Create "Set" Mealtimes As Often As You Can.

Do you remember when you were a kid, how mom had a set mealtime? Our family always ate at 5:30 p.m. Of course, sports and school activities disrupted this often as my brothers and I became teenagers, but having set mealtime whenever you can will help prevent unnecessary snacking.

Step 6: Avoid Mindless Eating.

Mindless eating can happen if you are bored or stressed, and it can also happen when you are happy! Think about your last graduation party or wedding. If you are like most people, you sampled this and that without even paying attention to how much you were eating. Try to put a plate together for yourself and just eat what's on your plate.

I run into this problem at food shows. There are thousands of vendors, and we're tasting hundreds of food samples. After the show, our first question is always, "Where should we have dinner?" There is absolutely no connection between our brains and stomachs. We just ate all this food, yet we are still hungry. Try putting food on a plate or napkin, even if you are at a cocktail party; it will help you to visualize what you are about to eat. You'll be less likely to overeat, and you'll be more likely to enjoy the food, too!

Are you ready to start applying some of these mindful eating practices?

According to Harvard University, the bottom line is that, "Combining behavioral strategies such as mindfulness training with nutrition knowledge can lead to healthful food choices that reduce the risk of chronic diseases, promote more enjoyable meal experiences, and support a healthy body image.[lxxii]"

What can be better than that?

Chapter 12 Summary:

- Mindfulness in eating involves slowing down and focusing solely on the act of eating, without distractions.
- Eating mindfully has numerous health benefits, including improved digestion and potentially aiding in weight management.
- Four key steps to mindful eating are outlined: Arriving at the Food, Awakening, Tuning into Your Body, and Service Around the Food.
- Arriving at the Food involves assessing the nutritional value and composition of the food on your plate.
- Awakening is the act of truly tasting and savoring your food, and paying attention to its flavors, textures, and aromas.
- Tuning into Your Body encourages slowing down and being aware of your body's signals of hunger and fullness.
- Practicing mindful eating habits while taking GLP-1 medications can help you to intuitively manage food choices, lose weight, regulate blood-sugar, and prepare for potential future transitions off the medication.
- Service Around the Food emphasizes the importance of creating a conducive environment for mindful eating, including sitting down, avoiding distractions, and making meals aesthetically pleasing.
- Additional tips include making meals last at least 20 minutes, establishing set meal times, and avoiding mindless eating.
- Combining m ndfulness with nutrition knowledge can lead to healthier food choices, enjoyable meal experiences, and improved body image

Chapter 12 Goals:

Nutrition: Clear your mind before every meal. While eating, remember to try to chew every bite 10-15 times.

Fitness: Stick with my recommendations and whatever you have added to your exercise regimen based on your personal interests.

Hydration: Continue aiming for 64 ounces of water a day.

Lasagna Rollups

This recipe makes 12 servings

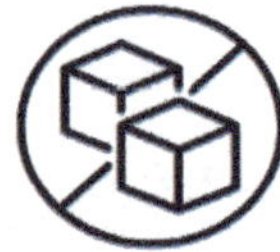

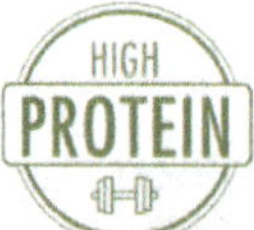

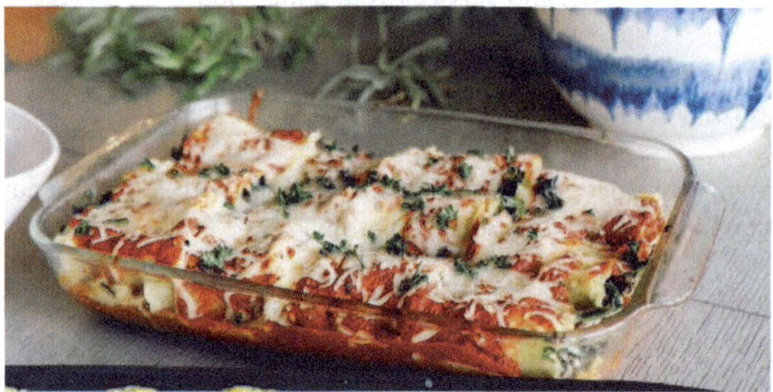

Ingredients

- 12 sheets lasagna noodles
- 1 lb. lean ground beef
- 1 cup skim-milk ricotta cheese
- 10 oz. frozen spinach, thawed
- 1 egg
- 1 cup part-skim mozzarella cheese
- 1/4 cup grated Parmesan cheese
- 1/4 cup mushrooms, minced
- 1 jar marina sauce
- 2 Tbsp. parsley, chopped

Directions

Preheat oven to 350 degrees F. In a pot, boil water, and cook lasagna noodles according to box directions. Drain and rinse with cool water and set aside. In a pan, cook ground beef until no longer pink. Drain additional liquid, and set aside.

In a medium bowl, mix ricotta cheese, spinach, egg, mozzarella, Parmesan, and mushrooms.

In a baking dish, cover bottom with marinara sauce, leaving some sauce to top pasta later. Lay noodles flat, spread 2 Tbsp. of mixture across noodle. Roll up noodle and mixture and place in baking dish.

In a medium bowl, mix ricotta cheese, spinach, egg, mozzarella, Parmesan, and mushrooms.

In a baking dish, cover bottom of dish with marinara sauce, leaving some sauce to top pasta later.

Lay noodles flat. Spread 2

2 Tbsp. of mixture across noodle. Roll up the noodle and mixture. Place in baking dish. Once completed, top roll ups with remaining marinara and additional mozzarella cheese. Bake 25-30 minutes. Top with parsley and enjoy!

CHAPTER 13: DIVING INTO DIGESTION

In our journey together so far, you have learned what your plate should look like at each meal and the Power of Five—protein, veggies, fruit, dairy, and whole grains. You have also learned how to limit added sugar and reduce your salt intake. And to make this ideal plate possible, you have learned some pretty cool strategies.

In this chapter, you will learn about the hot topic of gut health. This is a critical chapter for you if you are on weight-loss drugs. Common side effects of GLP-1s include nausea, vomiting, and diarrhea. These symptoms can be severe for some individuals and may lead to dehydration and electrolyte imbalances if not managed properly. So, in addition to keeping yourself hydrated as I have been challenging you to do throughout the book, learning how to balance your gut flora may help to lessen these uncomfortable symptoms.

The trend of gut health wellness, along with scientific discoveries over the past decade, has contributed to an interest in those trillions of bacteria hanging out in your gut; their community is called a microbiome. This is good news! This knowledge needs to get out there. But what "bugs" me about the media attention is that it causes confusion. I am excited to diffuse this confusion to the point where you can call yourself a gut health expert.

Good, healthy gut health does so much more than digesting your food; good gut health can help you lose weight, prevent type-2 diabetes, reduce your risk of heart disease and cancer, and even bolster your mood!

Consider this—you have 10 times more bacteria cells in your body than human cells!

I learned about gut health through personal experience, right at the brink of researchers discovering the many ways that a healthy gut affects overall well-being.

This was circa 2012 when my daughter Livi was five years old. She always complained of a bellyache before bed; I would just tell her to go to bed with a pillow on her tummy. One night, when complaining of a bellyache, she was in tears. I looked at her little belly and it was so distended! I immediately took her to the emergency room and soon after she was tested for lactose intolerance. Even though the doctor determined that she was not lactose intolerant, his advice was, "Just try giving her lactose-free milk." But, that didn't solve the problem.

We were so fortunate to visit Strong Memorial Hospital for a second opinion. We lucked out with a resident who was doing his PhD thesis on gut bacteria. This is the first time I had heard about prebiotics and probiotics. Turns out my daughter had gut dysbiosis; this is an imbalance of gut bacteria. She had recently been on antibiotics (which kills gut bacteria around the same time of Halloween—a time of year when most kids consume a lot of sugar (which also reduces any beneficial gut bacteria)!

I had to rebuild my daughter's gut. Since then, I have been guiding patients through the same process because as I have witnessed, many, many people have imbalanced gut flora.

Now, it's your turn to learn!

Prebiotics, Probiotics, and Your Microbiome

I'll begin by describing the community hanging out in your intestines and how they function:

Probiotics are beneficial bacteria, and prebiotics are food for these bacteria. Probiotics are found in certain food that you consume. One of the best sources of probiotics are **fermented foods** like apple cider vinegar, sauerkraut, yogurt, raw cheese, miso, kefir (it's like a smoothie but with a slightly more bitter taste), kombucha (a carbonated iced tea drink that comes in hundreds of flavors), kimchi (a spicy cabbage),and tempeh (fermented soy).

If you don't have enough probiotics, the side effects can include:

- digestive disorders
- skin issues such as eczema
- candida
- frequent colds and flus

By adding more probiotic foods into your diet, you could see all of the following health benefits:

- Improved digestion
- stronger immune system
- increased energy from production of vitamin B12
- better breath because probiotics destroy candida
- healthier skin because probiotics improve eczema and psoriasis

- reduced cold and flu symptoms
- healing from leaky gut and inflammatory bowel disease
- weight loss of maintenance

Also, a 2021 study of diabetic rats[lxxiii] revealed that the combination of GLP-1 medications and probiotics have a synergistic effect—this combination (along with resveratrol (found in red grapesdramatically increased the GLP-1 levels in the intestinal tissues.

I have had many patients ask me about probiotic pills. It does seem easier to pop a pill than try to incorporate foods with weird names into your diet, right? But, it doesn't have to be that difficult. I have a great smoothie recipe at the end of this chapter that incorporates kefir. Things like kefir and kombucha are sold already prepared for you! Popping a probiotic pill is not the answer, because stomach acids will often destroy them before they even get to your intestines. When you eat probiotic food, the food itself provides a protective armor that helps shield the probiotics (friendly bacteria.) It also speeds the transport out of the stomach and into your digestive tract.

To keep those probiotics alive, you need to be sure to consume prebiotics.The beneficial bacteria in your gut eat this fiber.

Some great prebiotics to include in your diet are dandelion greens, berries, onions, asparagus, bananas, legumes, barley, oats, apples, burdock root, flaxseeds, and seaweed.

When you incorporate more prebiotics and probiotics into your diet, you will have a very happy microbiome.

Try combining some prebiotics together with probiotics in your meals like berries and yogurt, miso soup with onions or garlic, or stir-fried tempeh and asparagus; this will have a dynamic effect. Also, the recipe section has some great dynamic duo combinations for you!

It is important to note that taking antibiotics can kill your friendly gut bacteria, so when you need to take an antibiotic, it is ultra-important to increase your consumption of probiotics and prebiotics.

The overall goal is to create and sustain a healthy gut microbiome.

Check out how a healthy gut benefits your body:

- lower risk of heart disease[lxxiv]
- healthier cholesterol level[lxxv]
- lower stress response[lxxvi lxxvii]
- better balance of hunger-stimulating hormones[lxxviii]
- better balance of estrogen, improving PMS and menopause and reducing risk of PCOS[lxxix]
- higher immune function[lxxx]
- lower risk for obesity and weight gain[lxxxi]
- lower inflammation and autoimmune reactions[lxxxii]

Fiber

We can't talk about gut health without talking about my fantastic friend—fiber. Eating foods high in dietary fiber can do so much more than keep you regular. It can lower your risk for heart disease, stroke, and diabetes, improve the health of your skin, and help you lose weight. It may even help prevent colon cancer.[lxxxiii]

Here's an analogy that I learned from Dr. Margaret Voss, who teaches nutritional biochemistry at Syracuse University. Your gut has this mucosa layer. This is a house for all your bacteria. Fiber builds this house. If there is no house for the bacteria, your bacteria will seep out because it has nowhere to go. This causes leaky gut syndrome, which leads to massive inflammation—the precursor to most chronic diseases.

I have mentioned fiber over one hundred times so far in this book because it is literally one of the most important things to consider when preventing chronic diseases.

In addition to aiding digestion and preventing constipation, fiber adds bulk to your diet,which is a key factor in both losing weight and maintaining a healthy weight. Adding bulk can help you feel full sooner. Because fiber stays in the stomach longer than other foods, that feeling of fullness will stay with you much longer, helping you eat less. High-fiber foods such as fruits and vegetables tend to be low in calories, so by adding fiber to your diet, it's easier to cut calories.

By regulating your blood sugar levels, fiber can help maintain your body's fat-burning capacity and avoid insulin spikes that leave you feeling drained and craving unhealthy foods. Eating plenty of fiber can also move fat through your digestive system faster so that less of it can be absorbed. And when you fill up on high-fiber foods, you'll also have more energy for exercising.

Emerging research also shows that fiber helps increase the diversity of friendly gut bacteria.[lxxxiv]

Remember that individuals up to age 50 should have between 25 and 38 grams of fiber each day, and people over the age of 50 should aim for 21 to 30 grams of fiber each day.

I again suggest for you to review the high-fiber food choices on pages 31-32. And at the end of the book that have a high-fiber icon. Here are some more tips:

- Fiber from fruit
  - Add fruit to your breakfast.
  - Keep fruits at your fingertips.
  - Replace dessert with fruit.
  - Eat whole fruits instead of drinking fruit juice.
  - Eat the peel when you can.
- Fiber from vegetables
  - Incorporate veggies into your cooking.
  - Bulk up soups and salads.
  - Don't leave out the legumes.
  - Sliced veggies make a great snack!
  - Eat the peel when you can.
- Fiber from whole grains
  - Start your day with fiber. Look for whole grain cereals. For example, switching your breakfast cereal from Corn Flakes to Bran Flakes can add an extra 6 g of fiber to your diet.
  - Replace white rice, bread, and pasta with brown rice and whole grain products. Experiment with wild rice, barley, whole-wheat pasta, and bulgur. Choose whole grain bread for toast and sandwiches.
  - Use whole wheat flour or oat flour and in your baking
  - Add ground flaxseed to your baking.

When it comes to packaged foods, labels are misleading, claiming a food is a "good source" of fiber if it delivers 10% of your daily dose of fiber—about 2.5 grams per serving. The terms "rich in," "high in," or "an excellent source of" fiber are allowed if the product contains 5 or more grams of fiber per serving. Your best bet for bread? Look for the words "100% whole wheat" or "100% whole grain" on the label and at least 3 grams of fiber per slice.

Keep in mind that the serving size can be tricky. For example, my patient Tim was so happy with his choice of bread because he thought he was getting 4 grams of fiber from the bread when he ate his sandwiches. He noticed that the amount of fiber on the label was 2 grams, so he figured two pieces of bread was 4 grams of fiber. What he didn't notice is that the serving size was two slices of bread, so unfortunately, he was only getting 2 grams of fiber from his sandwich.

Hydration

I have been giving you hydration challenges at the end of every chapter because water has so many health benefits.

Proper hydration is required for maintaining a healthy brain and energy levels, assuring healthy blood flow, proper kidney function, and proper sodium/potassium/electrolyte balance.

So, it probably comes to no surprise that water intake also plays a huge role in digestion.

Water helps improve the digestive process and is imperative in maintaining a healthy urinary tract and digestive system. Water is important to properly metabolize food. Drinking sufficient amounts of water will also help reduce constipation, which is actually the storage of waste in your body. You want to rid of that stuff!

Drinking sufficient amounts of water will help the body process and transport nutrients and excrete any waste products once they are metabolized.

Did you know that water can suppress appetite naturally and increases the body's ability to metabolize stored fat? Studies show that a decrease in water intake will cause fat deposits to increase, while an increase in water intake can actually reduce fat deposits.

For example, in a study published in *The Journal of Natural Science, Biology and Medicine*[lxxxv]researchers studied 50 overweight females and had them drink 500 milliliters (close to 17 ounces[lxxxvi]) of water 30 minutes before breakfast, lunch, and dinner. This was in addition to their regular water consumption, for eight consecutive weeks. The participants experienced a reduction in body weight, body fat, and body mass index. They also reported appetite suppression.

A 2016 mini-review[lxxxvii] found that drinking more water led to an increase in the metabolism of stored fat.

Your Gut and Your Mood

Did you know that there is thing called the gut-brain axis? This is a communication pathway between your gut and your brain. In fact, 95% of your serotonin (the happy hormone is produced in your gut! This neurotransmitter travels from your gut to your brain. If your gut microbiome is out of balance, you will not be manufacturing enough serotonin.

In fact, my patient Ally, was prescribed antidepressants for years; she survived on diet soda and a lot of chip-type snacks during her chaotic schedule as a teacher. We worked on rebalancing her gut health and she was able to get off her antidepressants.

She said, "I am happy for the first time in my life. And things that normally cause me intense stress and anxiety don't affect me anymore. It's amazing!"

Your Gut and Your Bone Health

Another thing I want to mention is that that your gut health can affect your bone mass![lxxxviii] Many of my patients with osteopenia or osteoporosis came to me knowing about the importance of calcium and vitamin D in bone health, but they don't know about vitamin K2. Vitamin K2 ensures that calcium is absorbed, which can increase your bone mass. While vitamin K2 can be found in food, it is also produced in a healthy gut.

I have seen numerous occasions where my elderly patients have improved bone mass by working on their gut health.

Concluding Thoughts

Do you see how your gut is an entire universe, and it directly impacts your overall health? Try getting in foods that have probiotics and foods that have prebiotics every day. Read your labels. Make sure you are meeting fiber requirements. Add grains, nuts and seeds to your diet. Add fruits and veggies for snacks. Maintain the hydration challenge of 64 ounces of water every day.

Chapter 12 Summary:

- Understanding the role of probiotics and prebiotics in gut health is essential not only to address uncomfortable gut-related side effects from taking GLP-1 medications, but also, for overall well-being.
- Incorporating probiotic-rich foods like fermented foods (kefir, yogurt, etc.) and prebiotic-rich foods (onions, bananas, etc.) into the diet can promote a healthy microbiome.
- Synergistic effects of GLP-1 medications and probiotics may offer promising avenues for improving gut health.
- Dietary sources of probiotics are preferable to probiotic pills due to their protective effects and higher survivability.
- Balancing probiotics and prebiotics in meals can have dynamic effects on gut health and overall health.
- During antibiotic use, increasing intake of probiotics and prebiotics is crucial for maintaining gut health.
- Beyond digestion, gut health influences various aspects of well-being, including heart health, immune function, mood, and bone health.
- Fiber plays a vital role in gut health by supporting the mucosa layer, preventing inflammation, and promoting regularity.
- Hydration is essential for proper digestion and overall health, with studies showing its benefits for weight loss and metabolism.
- Recognizing the gut-brain axis underscores the connection between gut health and mental well-being, highlighting the potential for gut health interventions to improve mood.
- Improving gut health can positively impact bone health by promoting vitamin K2 production, emphasizing the importance of gut health for bone density.

- Overall, your healthy food choices, increased water consumption and mindful eating habits improve gut health. And that can lengthen and enhance the quality of your life!

Goals:

Nutrition: Try some prebiotic and probiotic combinations at least three days a week.

Fitness: Keep up with your chosen exercise, whether jogging, cycling, dancing, or practicing yoga.

Hydration: Maintain the habit of drinking 64 ounces of water a day.

Probiotic Berry Smoothie
This recipe makes 1 serving

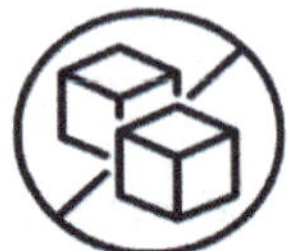
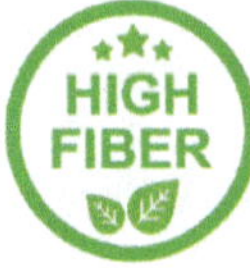

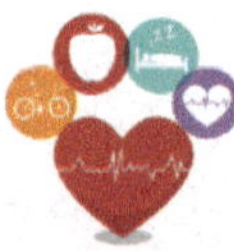
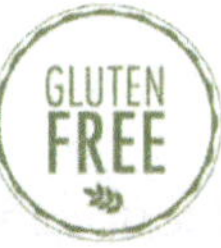

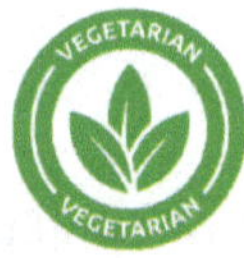

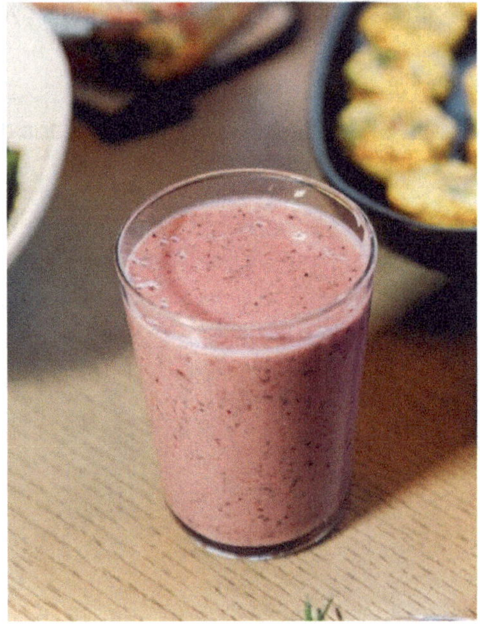

Ingredients

- 1 cup plain Lifeway Kefir
- 1/2 cup frozen mixed berries
- 1 banana
- 1 Tbsp. chia seeds
- Honey to taste

Directions

In a blender, blend kefir with mixed berries, banana and chia seeds until smooth. Sweeten with honey to taste. Pour into a glass and enjoy!

CHAPTER 14: SUSTAINING YOUR PROGRESS

Congratulations! You did it! You have taken the journey required to gain a healthier lifestyle. But, most importantly, you have gained the knowledge you need to help treat and prevent chronic conditions. And you have learned valuable strategies for maintaining weight loss whether or not you continue with GLP-1 medications. Remember that knowledge is power.

The journey to a continued healthy and happy quality of life does not stop here. If you fall off the healthy lifestyle staircase, start back up, even if it is baby steps.

This chapter will review all the chapters—so consider it an abbreviated version of the entire book. It also includes guidance on creating sustainable goals.

Nutrition Education and GLP-1 Receptor Agonists for Weight Loss Success

In Chapter 1, you learned about the role of GLP-1 (glucagon-like peptide-1) receptor agonists in managing type-2 diabetes and aiding weight loss. GLP-1 receptor agonists like Byetta®, Victoza®, Trulicity®, Ozempic®, and Mounjaro® mimic the natural hormone GLP-1, which regulates blood sugar, appetite, and has cardiovascular benefits. Popular options include tirzepatide (Mounjaro®), which mimics GLP-1 and GIP hormones, and semaglutide (Ozempic®, Wegovy®), which mimics GLP-1 alone. Nutrition education complements these medications by promoting healthy habits like balanced eating, exercise, and behavior modification, enhancing the effectiveness of GLP-1 receptor agonists in achieving long-term health and weight management.

The Power of Five

This is the foundation of healthy living. Make sure that every meal has whole grains, protein, vegetables, fruit, and low-fat dairy. Vegans can of course skip the dairy, but make sure you are getting good sources of calcium from leafy greens, for example. Plus, if this is you, consider a mineral supplement, as well as a vitamin B12 supplement.

When it comes to the Power of Five, I like to see lots of vegetables; so look at your plate—aim for half of it to be vegetables (more on this in a few paragraphs).

Crazy for Carbohydrates

Hopefully, you are like many of my patients and have recovered from carb-phobia, recognizing that carbs are a good thing if they're from the rainbow's "pot of gold." The pot of gold is filled with fiber-rich vegetables, whole grains and fruits. If you have yet to try a new grain, like farro, I encourage you to tryone. You will be amazed by how satisfying it is.

The trick with carbs is to refuse to let the sneaky leprechaun take control of your diet by slipping you refined carbs. It could be doughnuts at the conference table or the cookies your neighbor constantly brings to you. These goodies are loaded with added sugar, which is extremely addictive! So, kindly refuse or take a tiny serving.

If you can, try to remember the number 45! This is how many grams of carbs you want to try to consume at each meal.

And then there's fiber number—so important! You want to aim for 7-10 grams of fiber per meal.

Powerful Protein

Remember that protein is essential because it carries nutrients to your cells and provides structure for every single organ, your bones, muscles, and skin!

But, the problem with the Standard American Diet is that people don't eat enough plant protein and tend to eat most of their protein at dinner. You can refer to pages 38-39 for plant protein ideas.

You really want to spread your protein consumption throughout the day because if you eat too much protein at one meal, it will store as fat!

Your goal should be 15-30 grams of protein per meal.

Facts about Fat

Fat is not bad; your brain needs it! You also need fat to be able to absorb fat-soluble vitamins like vitamins A, D, E, and K. It's important to consume mostly unsaturated fats while limiting saturated fat and really limiting trans fats. Trans fat lurks in packaged food, pastries, and anything fried!

Fill Up on Fruits and Vegetables

Remember my tips to make sure you get your veggies in every meal. These ideas are to help you enjoy vegetables and to not get bored of them. Try getting all of the colors of the rainbow in your vegetable selections. Each color represents different antioxidants, which help prevent free radicals from taking up residence in your cells. Vegetables will

Remember that frozen vegetables are just as healthy as fresh vegetables! Keep your meals interesting by having a cold veggie and a warm veggie at each meal. And explore spices to enhance the flavor of vegetables and try different cooking methods like roasting and grilling.

Fruit is good for you too and loaded with antioxidants. Fruit is nature's candy. Blueberries are my number one fruit recommendation!

Food Shopping and Meal Planning

Just like almost everything, planning helps you succeed! Plan your shopping day. Take inventory of what you have in your fridge, freezer, spice rack, and pantry. Choose some recipes you'd like to try for the week and list the ingredients you don't have. Take into consideration the Power of Five when exploring meal ideas. Speaking of ideas, Theme Nights make meals so fun!

It's helpful to keep certain items on hand in your fridge, freezer, and pantry (see pages 77-80.) This will make food shopping quicker and less stressful.

Shop with a list and stick to the perimeter of the store. This makes you a smart consumer and helps you save money in the process. And don't go shopping when you are hungry! Have a snack before you go to prevent impulse shopping.

Sneaky Sugar and Sodium

Try to watch your sodium and sugar consumption. Keep in mind that your saltshaker is not where your overconsumption of sodium comes from—it's packaged food. Soup, jarred sauces, frozen meals, and deli meats are common culprits. Look for "low sodium" marketing on these packaged foods.

When it comes to sugar, limit "added sugar." This is what will spike your blood sugar levels. Women should have no more than 24 grams of added sugar a day and men should have no more than 36 grams of added sugar a day.

All food manufacturers are required to have "added sugar" on their labels now. For things that don't have labels, like soda fountain drinks, don't let healthy-sounding drinks like "mango iced tea" fool you; they are loaded with sugar too. Choose water or an unsweetened seltzer, unsweetened iced tea or unsweetened iced coffee.

Upgrading Breakfast and Snacks

In this chapter, we talked about prioritizing breakfast. Study after study has proven that a hearty breakfast (a protein-fiber combo produces so many amazing outcomes. Not just weight loss; we're talking better concentration and balanced blood-sugar levels, and statistically speaking, even a higher likelihood of getting a promotion at your job!

I think it's important to have a healthy snack when you have a big gap between meals. Again, a protein-fiber combo will help keep you satisfied until your next meal

and will also stabilize your blood-sugar levels. Good examples are nut butter and veggies, a handful of raw nuts with an apple, hummus and carrots, or a cheese stick and some berries.

Sleep Essentials

Quality sleep is essential for your diet. If your sleep is not ideal, you will crave high-sugar and high-fat foods. Sleep is like a battery pack: You recharge your cellphone every night. You should do the same with your body. So, invest in some blackout shades; declutter your room; unglue yourself from your devices a few hours before bed; avoid sugar and alcohol before bed. You can trying setting an alarm for bedtime just like you do to wake up. Aim for 7-9 hours of *quality* sleep!

Dining Out

You will be able to manage your weight better with your own prepared meals, but, it is possible to dine out healthfully. Remember the food preparation words to avoid (au gratin, fried, battered, crispy, creamy, glazed, pan fried, cheesy, loaded, fritter, buttery, bisque). Keep in mind that you can substitute an unhealthy side dish that comes with your meal for a healthier side dish. Eat slowly; put your fork down between bites. Enjoy your company. With meals that are larger portions than the sizes you learned in this book, bring home some of it. Leftovers are a beautiful thing.

Eating Mindfully

The process of eating mindfully will help you tune into what you are eating and how it makes you feel. Step one is Arriving at your food. When food comes into your space (whether it's brought there by you, a waiter, a family member, whomever), take 30 seconds to assess it. The next step is Awakening. This is when you take the first bite of your food. Chew the food slowly; actually taste your food. The third step is Tuning into your Body—how does the food make your body feel? AYou also want the Service around your food to be conducive to healthy eating.

Meal times should be special; you are nourishing your body. We are all busy; we can't always have a sit-down meal with beautiful placemats and lit candles, but please carve yourself out at least 15-20 minutes for meals and sit down! Let your body know this is time for fueling. You have learned to put away your cell phone and pay attention to your food.

Diving into Digestion

The health of your gut symbolizes your overall health.

You have learned the importance of prebiotics and probiotics. They keep the healthy bacteria in your gut thriving. Fermented foods (miso, kefir, kombucha, sauerkraut, yogurt, raw cheese are the best sources of probiotics. Prebiotics (high-fiber containing foods like oats, apples, barley, and flaxseeds) feed your probiotics, keeping them alive.

In addition to feeding probiotics, high-fiber foods help build the mucosa layer that houses all the bacteria in your gut. If that layer isn't built well, bacteria will seep out; this is how leaky gut syndrome develops, which causes inflammation, and inflammation is the precursor for most diseases.

Goal Setting

So, now that you know how to eat healthier, what are your personal goals?

Create short-term goals first. What do you want to accomplish today? Maybe you want to shop for frozen vegetables, so you always have them on hand. Or, maybe you want to try replacing one of your red meat meals with fish. Or maybe you want to start by drinking more water!

Then, think about what you want to accomplish in a year. Maybe you have a goal weight. Do you want to lower your blood pressure? Be specific—how many pounds do you want to lose? Be realistic.

Losing weight will automatically reduce your likelihood of almost all chronic diseases. You will have more energy to keep up with your kids. You will have more zest for life!

What is your "Why?" What inspired you to want to eat healthier?

Set these goals and maintain them.

Life is like a chain. There are links that come up that are not conducive to maintaining a healthy lifestyle...good things like weddings, celebrations, and vacations are links that may not be the best for your health 145goals, and there are bad things too like job loss or breakups that may result in unhealthy nutrition habits. But, hey, there are more links ahead. Be gentle with yourself and move to the next link.

Get support

I am rooting for you, and so is the entire Kelly's Choice team! If you want extra support in maintaining your health goals, contact us at kellyschoice.org. Our talented Registered Dietitians are available to meet with you virtually. Most insurance policies cover our services.

For daily tips and nutrition advice, keep in touch with us on
Facebook (https://www.facebook.com/KChoiceLLC)
LinkedIn (https://www.linkedin.com/in/kellyschoice/)
Instagram (kellyschoice_nutrition).

RECIPES TO TRY

Apple With Almond Butter

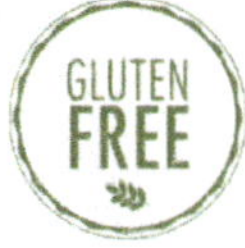

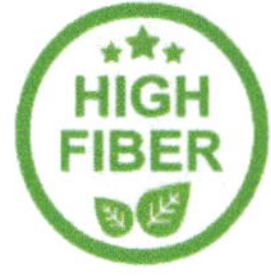

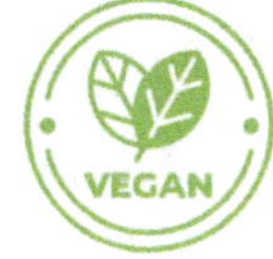

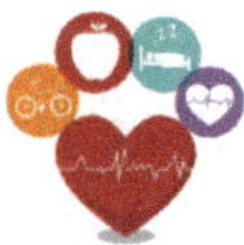

This recipe makes 1 serving

Ingredients

- 1 apple
- 1 Tbsp almond butter.

Directions

1. Core and cut apples into slices
2. Place almond butter into a small bowl.
3. Dip apples into almond butter and enjoy.

Asian Chicken Lettuce Wraps

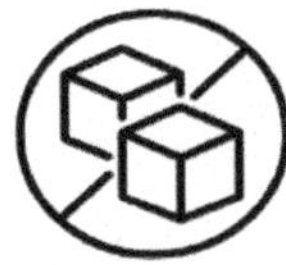

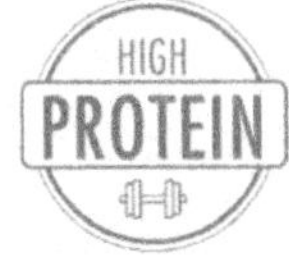

This recipe makes 3 servings

Ingredients

Sauce

- 1 Tbsp. soy sauce
- 1 Tbsp. Hoisin sauce
- 1/2 Tbsp. sesame oil
- 1/2 Tbsp. honey
- 1/3 Tbsp. rice vinegar
- 1/2 tsp. garlic powder

Chicken Stir-Fry

- 1/2 Tbsp. avocado oil
- 300 g ground chicken
- 1/2 onion, minced
- 1/2 garlic clove, minced
- 1/2 cup diced red bell pepper
- 12 leaves of butter lettuce
- 1/4 cup crushed peanuts for topping
- 1/4 cup chopped green onion

Directions

1. Whisk together sauce ingredients until evenly mixed.
2. Heat a medium or large skillet with avocado oil on high heat.
3. Sauté the ground chicken. Once it starts to brown, add the onions and garlic.
4. Once the onions are translucent, add the diced red bell pepper and cook for 5 minutes, or until soft.
5. Add the sauce mixture into the pan with the chicken and vegetables, and simmer on low heat for 2 minutes.

Baked Chicken and Vegetable Fajitas

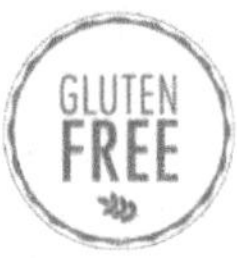

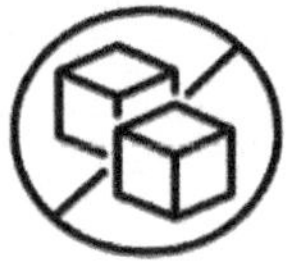
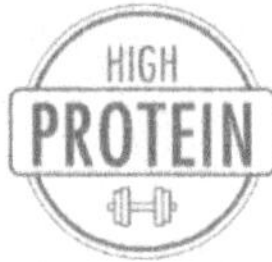

This recipe makes 20 servings

Ingredients

- 5 pounds skinless chicken breast
- 5 Tbsp. ground chili powder
- 7.5 cans drained and rinsed corn
- 5 tsp. garlic powder
- 10 Tbsp. extra- virgin olive oil
- 5 large yellow onions
- 5 medium red bell peppers
- 1 lime, sliced
- 3.75 tsp. salt
- 40 medium soft corn tortillas

Directions

1. Preheat oven to 400 degrees and spray baking sheet with cooking spray.
2. Slice chicken breast into thin slices and place in bowl.
3. Add extra virgin olive oil, chili powder, and salt into bowl with chicken.
4. Add sliced bell pepper and sliced yellow onion to a bowl.
5. Once all ingredients are evenly mixed, transfer mixture to baking sheet and spread evenly.
6. Place baking sheet in oven and cook for 15 minutes.
7. Turn on broiler for 5 minutes and allow veggies to begin to brown and ensure chicken is cooked through.
8. Put drained corn and cooked ingredients into bowl and mix all together.
9. Serve mixture with corn tortillas and side of lime, and optional side bowl of salsa and side of cilantro for a garnish.

Barley and Vegetable Soup

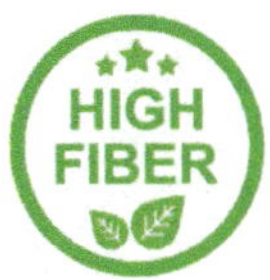

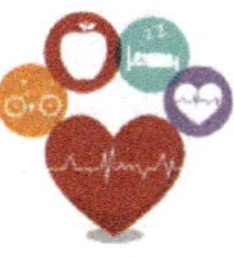
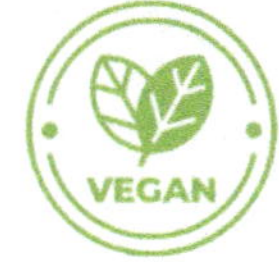

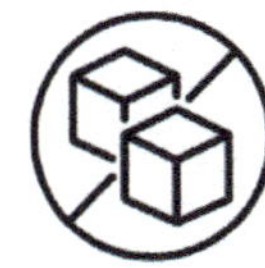

This recipe makes 4 servings

Ingredients

- 1 cup pearl barley, rinsed
- 6 cups vegetable broth
- 2 Tbps. olive oil
- 1 onion, diced
- 2 carrots, diced
- 2 celery stalks, diced
- 3 cloves garlic, minced
- 1 can (14 oz) diced tomatoes
- 1 tsp. dried thyme
- 1 tsp. dried rosemary
- Salt and pepper to taste
- 2 cups chopped spinach or kale
- Fresh parsley, for garnish
- Lemon wedges, for serving

Directions

1. In a large pot, heat olive oil over medium heat. Add diced onion, carrots, and celery. Sauté for 5-7 minutes, or until vegetables are softened.
2. Add minced garlic and sauté for an additional 1-2 minutes, until fragrant.
3. Stir in pearl barley and cook for 1-2 minutes, allowing the barley to toast slightly.
4. Pour in vegetable broth and diced tomatoes with their juices. Add dried thyme and rosemary. Season with salt and pepper to taste.
5. Bring the soup to a boil, then reduce heat to low. Cover and simmer for 30-40 minutes, or until the barley is tender.
6. Stir in chopped spinach or kale and cook for an additional 5 minutes, until greens are wilted.
7. Adjust seasoning if needed. Serve hot, garnished with fresh parsley and a squeeze of lemon juice.

Beef and Shitake Stir-Fry

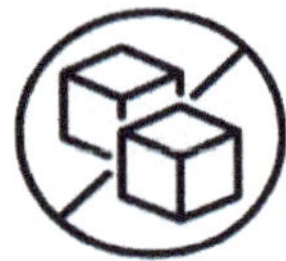
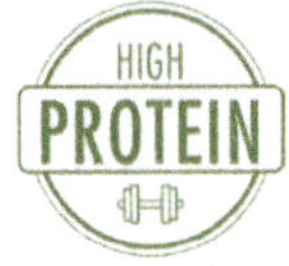

This recipe makes 4 servings

Ingredients

- 1 lb. beef strips
- 8 oz. shiitake mushrooms, sliced
- 1/4 cup soy sauce
- 2 tbsp. oyster sauce
- 3 cloves garlic, minced
- 1 tsp. ginger, grated
- 2 tbsp. sesame oil
- 1 cup broccoli florets
- 2 bell peppers, sliced

Directions

1. In a bowl, mix soy sauce, oyster sauce, garlic, and ginger to create the sauce.
2. Heat sesame oil in a wok or large pan over high heat.
3. Add beef strips and stir-fry until browned. Remove from the pan.
4. Stir-fry mushrooms, broccoli, and bell peppers until tender.
5. Return the beef to the pan, add the sauce, and toss everything together until heated through.

Black Bean Brownies

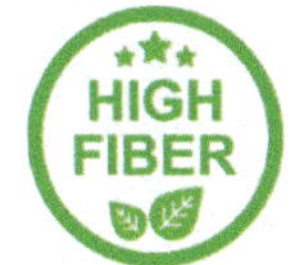

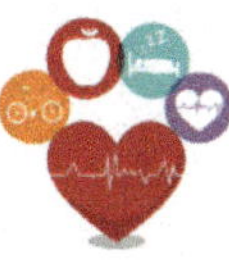
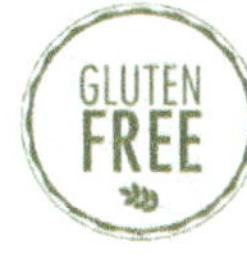

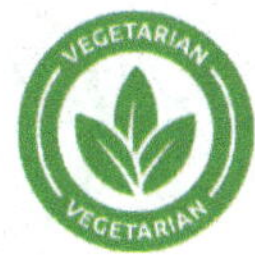

This recipe makes 16 squares

Ingredients

- Non-stick cooking spray
- .1 15 oz. can black beans, rinsed and drained
- 3 large eggs
- 3 Tbsp. unsweetened applesauce
- 1 tsp. vanilla extract
- 1/2 cup packed brown sugar
- 1/3 cup cocoa powder
- 1/2 cup chocolate, peanut butter, or butterscotch chips

Directions

1. Preheat oven to 350 degrees Fahrenheit. Spray a 9-inch square baking dish with non-stick cooking spray.
2. In a large bowl, use a fork to whisk eggs, applesauce, and vanilla. Add the beans, and mash with a fork until they are barely noticeable (you can put these ingredients in a blender or food processor too).
3. Stir the sugar and the cocoa into the bean and egg mixture. If using the chips, mix those in.
4. Pour batter into prepared baking dish. Bake until knife inserted in center comes out clean, about 25-30 minutes.
5. Allow to cool completely, then cut into 16 squares.

Blueberry Watermelon Salad

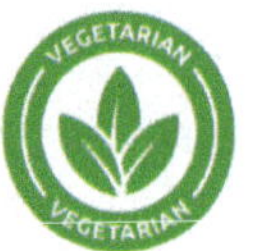

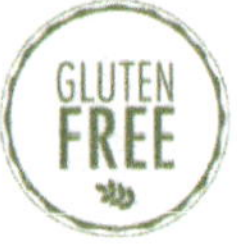

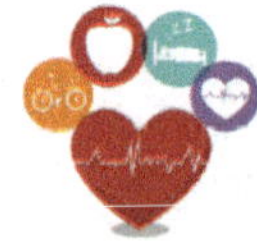

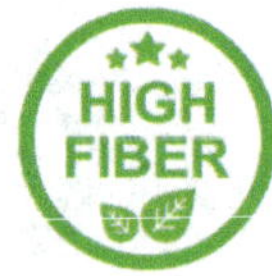

This recipe makes 4 servings

Ingredients

- 1/2 cup reduced-fat feta cheese
- 1 ½ cup blueberries
- 1 ½ cup sliced cucumbers
- 3 cups watermelon, cubed or balled
- 1 Tbsp. lime juice
- 2 Tbsp. mint leaves
- 3 Tbsp. olive oil
- Salt and pepper, to taste

Directions

1. In a mixing bowl, stir together blueberries, cucumbers, watermelon, and mint leaves.
2. In a separate small bowl, whisk together lime juice, olive oil, salt, and pepper.
3. Drizzle dressing over the fruit/cucumber mix. Toss to coat.
4. Top with feta and serve.

Butternut Squash & Apple Breakfast Hash

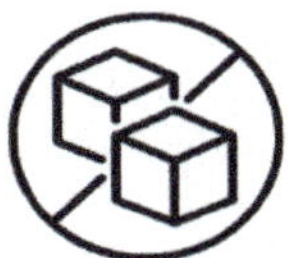
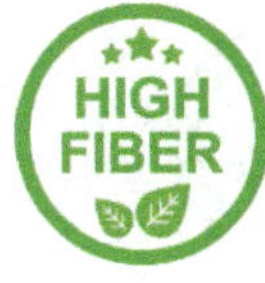

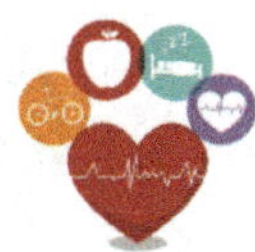
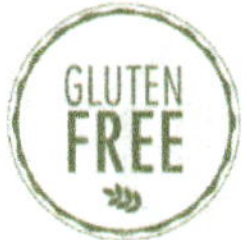

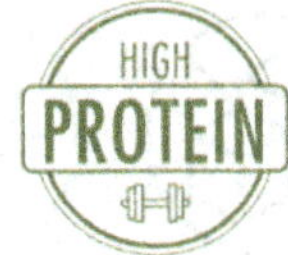

This recipe makes 4 servings

Ingredients

- 1.5 Tbsp. olive oil
- 3 Tbsp. water
- 1 onion
- 1 medium apple
- 1 small butternut squash
- 12 oz. 95% lean ground turkey or chicken
- 3 cups kale
- 1/2 tsp. salt
- 1/2 tsp. dried sage
- 1/4 tsp. garlic powder
- 1/4 tsp. red pepper flakes

Directions

1. Add olive oil to large skillet, and turn stove to medium-high heat.
2. Peel, de-seed, and chop the onion and butternut squash to bite sized pieces, and sauté for 8-10 minutes.
3. Dice the apple and add it to the skillet along with 3 Tbsp. of water. Cook for 5 minutes.
4. Push the veggie mixture to the side of the skillet and add in meat. Cook for 5-6 minutes, breaking up the meat into smaller pieces.
5. Mix together meat and vegetables.
6. Place kale on top of the hash before covering the skillet with a lid. Allow kale to cook for 1-2 minutes. Mix the hash again and add in salt, dried sage, garlic powder, and red pepper flakes.

Butternut Squash Salad

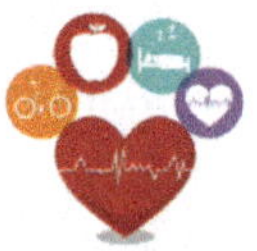
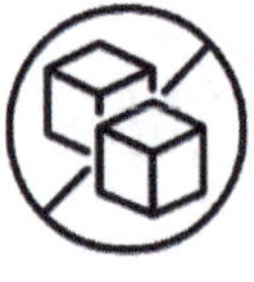
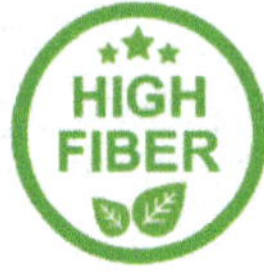

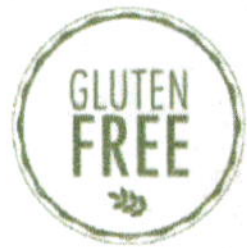

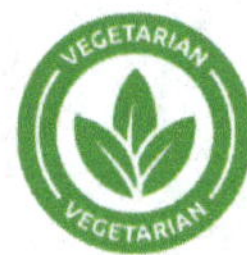

This recipe makes 4 servings

Ingredients

- 1 butternut squash
- 2 Tbsp. olive oil
- 1 Tbsp. maple syrup
- 1/2 tsp. salt
- 1/2 tsp. black pepper
- 3/4 cup apple cider vinegar
- 4 oz. baby arugula
- 1/2 cup walnut halves
- 3/4 cup parmesan cheese

Directions

1. Preheat oven to 400 degrees F.
2. Place squash on baking sheet and toss with olive oil and maple syrup. Roast for 15-20 minutes.
3. While the squash is roasting, add apple cider vinegar to a small saucepan and bring a boil over medium heat. Cook for 6 to 8 minutes until the cider is reduced to 1/4 cup. Turn off the heat and mix in black pepper.
4. Place arugula, roasted squash, walnuts, and cheese. Pour olive oil, salt, black pepper, and apple cider in the bowl and mix.

Chicken-Broccoli-Rice Bake

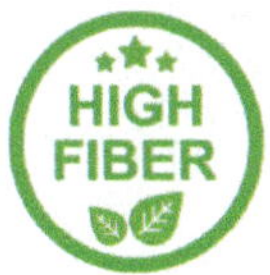

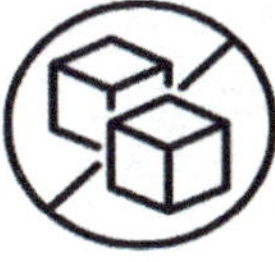
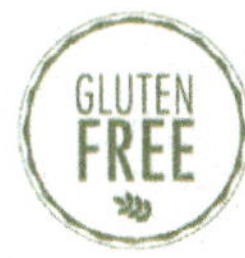

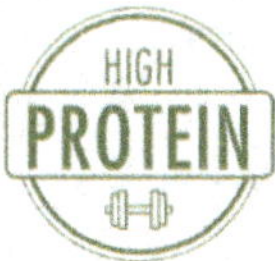

This recipe makes 4 servings

Ingredients

- 3.5 cups of water
- 1.5 cups of brown rice
- 2 chicken breasts chopped in small cubes
- 1 cup of sliced mushrooms
- 1 can of lite coconut milk
- 2 cups of broccoli florets
- 1 cup of low-fat cheddar cheese
- 1 tsp. of sea salt
- 2 Tbsp. olive oil
- 1 tsp. Italian seasoning
- Ground pepper to taste

Directions

1. Combine the rice, 1/2 teaspoon of sea salt, 1 Tbsp. olive oil, and 3 cups of water in a pot. Bring to a boil. Once boiling, cover and reduce to a simmer for 30-35 minutes. You can do this quicker with a rice cooker or instant pot!
2. 15 minutes prior to the rice finishing, add chicken to a deep pan or Dutch oven, and pan fry for 10-15 minutes over medium heat. Add the mushrooms and sauté for 2 minutes. If the chicken or mushrooms are sticking, add a couple tablespoons of water.
3. 5 minutes before the rice is finished, preheat oven to 350 degrees F. Add remaining 1/2 cup of water to a pot with a steamer basket. Bring to a boil. Place broccoli in basket, cover, and steam for 3 minutes.
4. When rice is finished, mix in pan with chicken and mushrooms. Toss in broccoli.
5. Mix in coconut milk, remaining sea salt, Italian seasoning, and cheese.
6. Transfer to a casserole dish and add ground pepper to taste.
7. Bake for 15 minutes.

Chicken Caprese Kebabs

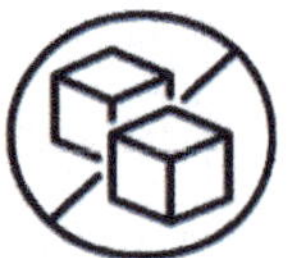
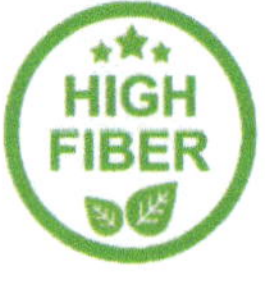

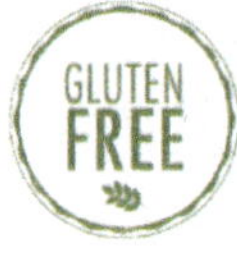

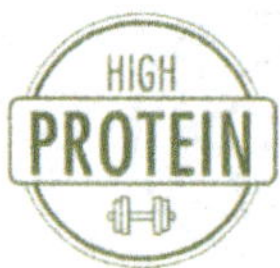

This recipe makes 4 servings

Ingredients

- 2 lb. boneless, skinless chicken breasts
- 1-pint grape tomatoes
- 1 Tbsp. olive oil (for the chicken and tomatoes)
- 1/3 cup olive oil (for the pesto)
- 2 tsp. rosemary
- One 8 oz. package of low-fat mozzarella, cut into cubes
- Salt and freshly ground black pepper
- 4 Tbsp. balsamic glaze
- 2 cups fresh basil leaves
- 3 Tbsp. parmesan cheese, shredded
- 2 Tbsp. walnuts, chopped
- 2 tsp. garlic, minced
- Skewers for grilling

Directions

1. Soak skewers in cold water for at least 20 minutes before grilling.
2. Preheat grill over medium-high heat.
3. Thread chicken and tomatoes onto skewers.
4. Brush both sides with olive oil and rosemary, and sprinkle with salt and pepper.
5. Grill kebabs about 5 minutes per side, or until cooked all the way through.
6. While kebabs are grilling, blend or pulse basil, parmesan, nuts, and garlic several times.
7. Add salt and pepper, to taste. Slowly pour in olive oil and blend.
8. Thread one mozzarella cube onto each end of the skewer; drizzle pesto and balsamic glaze over kebabs and enjoy!

Chickpeas, Black-Eyed Peas, & Rice Vegetable Blend

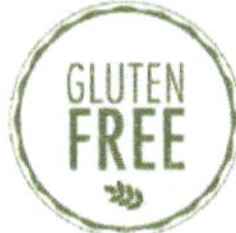

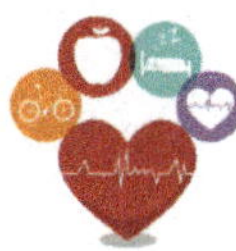
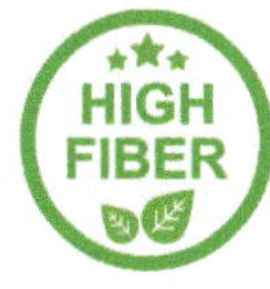

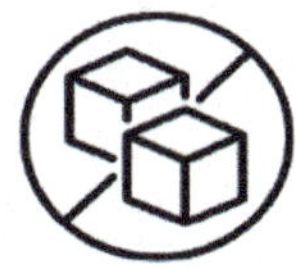
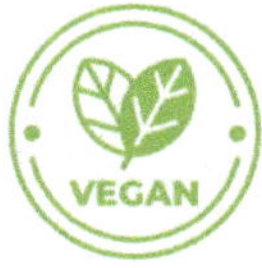

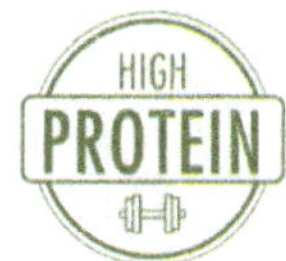

This recipe makes 10 servings

Ingredients

- 5 cups of uncooked long- grain brown rice
- 10 cups of water
- Three 15.5 oz. cans of chickpeas
- Three 15.5 oz. of black-eyed peas
- Three 14.5 oz. cans of tomatoes
- 4 Tbsp. of extra virgin olive oil
- 3 chopped onions
- Three 12 oz. bags chopped spinach
- 3 Tbsp. of garlic powder
- Salt and pepper to taste

Directions

1. Combine 5 cups of uncooked rice and 10 cups of water in a saucepan, and bring to a boil.
2. Turn heat to low and cover with a lid. Simmer for 45 minutes.
3. While rice is cooking, drain all 3 cans of chickpeas and rinse.
4. In a large saucepan, combine chickpeas, black-eyed peas, and 2 cups of water. Bring to a medium-low heat and simmer for 25 minutes.
5. Drain 3 cans of tomatoes.
6. In a large skillet, add 4 tbsp. of extra virgin olive oil, tomatoes, onions, spinach, and garlic powder. Sauté on medium-low heat for 10 minutes. Veggies should be soft when done.
7. Combine rice, chickpeas, black-eyed peas, and vegetables in a large bowl.

Cottage Cheese & Fruit

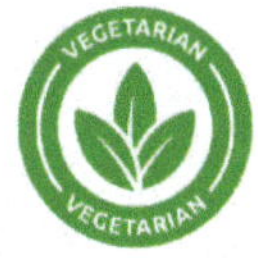

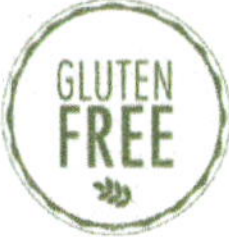

This recipe makes 1 serving

Ingredients

- 1/2 cup of low -fat cottage cheese
- 1/4 cup of raspberries or fruit of your choice

Directions

1. Put serving of cottage cheese in a bowl.
2. Place raspberries on top of cottage cheese.
3. Add some honey on top if desired. Enjoy!

Cranberry Orange Breakfast Millet

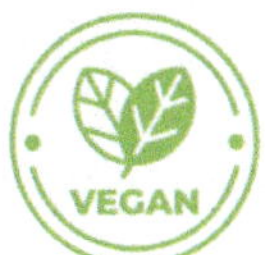

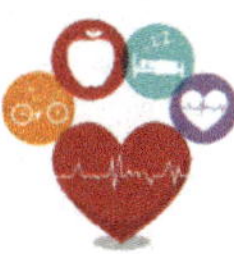
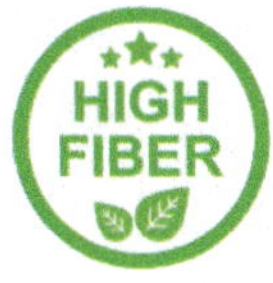

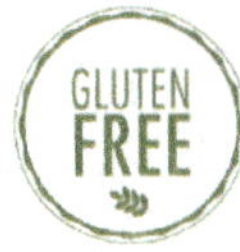

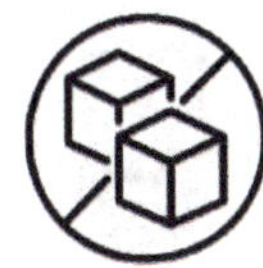

This recipe makes 2 servings

Ingredients

- 1/2 cup millet
- 1 cup coconut milk
- 1/4 cup chopped walnuts
- 1/2 tsp. cinnamon
- Zest of one orange
- 1 cup fresh cranberries
- Drizzle of honey or maple syrup (optional))

Directions

1. Toast dry millet and walnuts in a pot over low heat for 3-5 minutes.
2. Add coconut milk and bring to a boil.
3. Add all other ingredients and reduce to a simmer for 25 minutes.
4. Drizzle with honey or maple syrup for some sweetness.

Cucumber Tomato Salad

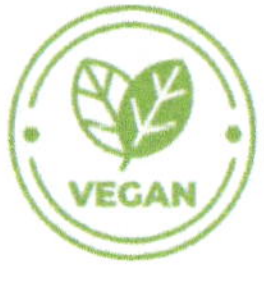

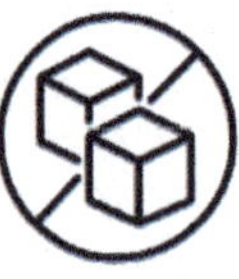

This recipe makes 1 serving

Ingredients

- 1 large cucumber
- 2 large tomatoes
- 1/2 small sweet onion
- 1/4 cup fresh basil
- 3 Tbsp. red wine vinegar
- 1 Tbsp. olive oil
- 1 medium garlic clove, minced
- Black pepper to taste

Directions

1. Peel and slice cucumber.
2. Dice tomatoes into 1/2 inch pieces.
3. Cut onion into 1/4 inch wide slices.
4. Combine in large bowl.
5. Whisk remaining ingredients together in a separate bowl and drizzle over salad.
6. Toss to mix.

Delicata Squash and Pear Soup

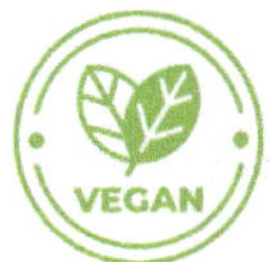

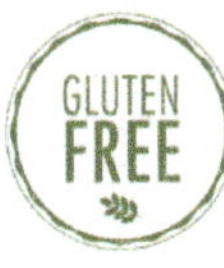

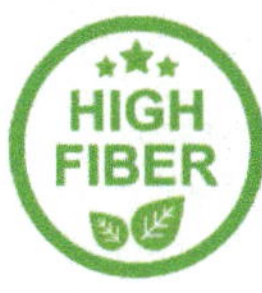

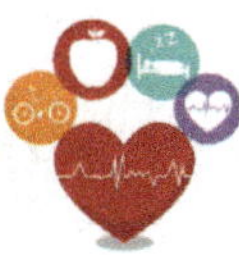

This recipe makes 2 servings

Ingredients

- 3 or 4 delicata squash, chopped and seeded
- 2 pears, cored and chopped
- Water-to cover
- Pinch of salt
- 1/2 tsp. basil
- 1/2 tsp. sage
- 1/2 tsp. nutmeg
- 1 Tbsp. olive oil

Directions

1. Place squash and pear in large pot.
2. Cover with just enough water to cover squash/pear mixture.
3. Place lid on pot and bring to a boil.
4. Add a pinch of salt, a dash of olive oil, and your herbs.
5. Cook on medium heat for 20-30 minutes, or until squash is tender.
6. Once cooked, use a hand-held blender or food processor to puree to a smooth and rich consistency.

Easy Egg Custard

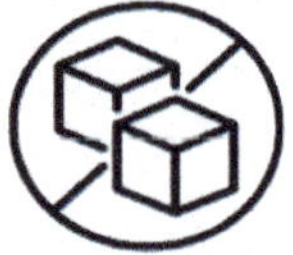
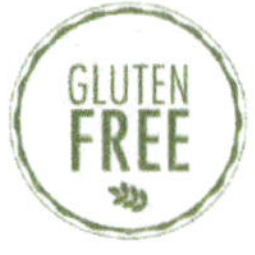

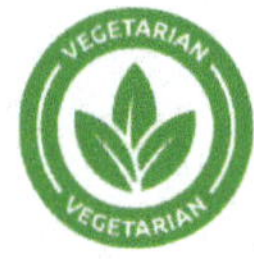

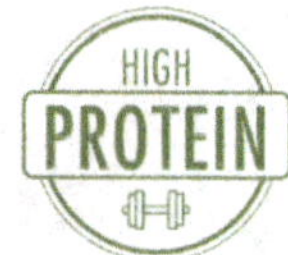

This recipe makes 6 servings

Ingredients

- 2 cups whole milk
- 2 large eggs
- 2 large egg yolks
- 1/3 cup sugar
- 1 tsp. vanilla extract
- Ground nutmeg

Directions

1. Preheat oven to 300 degrees F. Place 6 4-oz ovenproof ramekin in a deep baking pan.
2. In a saucepan, bring milk to a simmer over medium-low heat.
3. In a separate bowl, whisk together eggs, yolks, sugar, and vanilla. Slowly pour warm milk into egg mixture, whisking gently.
4. Pour mixture through strainer into the ramekins, then sprinkle with nutmeg.
5. Fill baking pan halfway with hot water.
6. Bake until just set (about 30-35 minutes).
7. Let custard cool in water bath for 2 hours before serving.

Egg Drop Soup

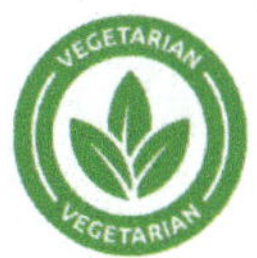

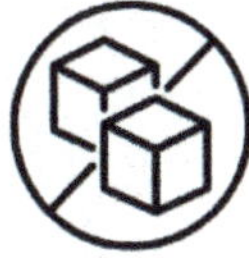
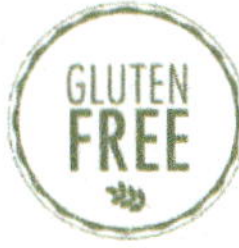

This recipe makes 6 servings

Ingredients

- 4 cups reduced sodium vegetable stock
- 1 cup sliced mushrooms (canned, fresh, or frozen)
- 3/4 cup corn (canned, fresh, or frozen)
- 1 Tbsp. light soy sauce
- 1 Tbsp. cornstarch
- 3 eggs, lightly beaten
- 3 green onions, chopped

Directions

1. Pour stock into medium pot, reserving 1/4 cup to the side.
2. Add mushrooms, corn, and soy sauce to the pot. Bring to a boil.
3. Whisk cornstarch in reserved stock. Set aside.
4. Lightly beat eggs. Set aside.
5. Once stock is boiling, lower to a simmer. Add cornstarch mixture.
6. While continuously stirring stock, slowly add eggs. This will create the egg ribbons.
7. Top with green onions and serve hot.

Greek Chicken Couscous Bowl with Tzatziki Sauce

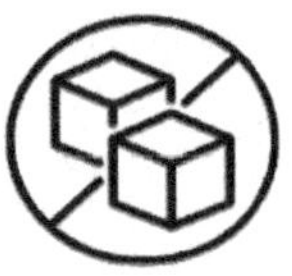
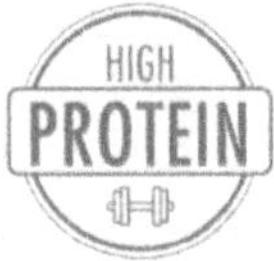

This recipe makes 2 servings

Ingredients

Chicken

- 1/2 tsp. dried rosemary
- 1/2 tsp. ground black pepper
- 1/2 tsp. salt
- 1/2 tsp. dried oregano
- 1/2 tsp. garlic powder
- 1/2 tsp. onion powder
- 1/2 tsp. sea salt
- 1/4 tsp. ground coriander
- 1/8 tsp. ground cardamom
- 2 skinless, boneless chicken breasts
- 2 Tbsp. vegetable oil
- 1 lemon, juice

Tzatziki Sauce

- 2 cups grated cucumber
- 1.5 cups plain Greek yogurt
- 2 Tbsp. olive oil
- 2 Tbsp. fresh dill
- 1 Tbsp. lemon juice
- 1 clove garlic, minced

Couscous

- 1 package of instant couscous
- 1.5 cup water or low-sodium chicken broth

Directions

For chicken:

1. Preheat oven to 350 degrees F.
2. Combine vegetable oil and all chicken seasonings in a bowl; drizzle evenly over the chicken breasts.
3. Bake chicken for 25-30 minutes. Once baked, cut into strips or 1-inch cubes.
4. While the chicken bakes, prepare the Tzatziki sauce and couscous.

For Tzatziki Sauce:

1. Grate 1 cucumber using the large holes on your grater. Remove excess moisture by lightly squeezing over the sink; set in bowl.
2. Add the remaining ingredients to the bowl and mix. Let the mixture sit for at least 5 minutes.

For Couscous:

1. Bring water or chicken broth to a boil. Remove from heat and pour in instant couscous. Let sit for 5 minutes, or until all the liquid is absorbed. Use a fork to fluff the couscous.

Assemble chicken, couscous, and toppings of your choice on a plate or in a bowl. Top with Tzatziki and enjoy!

Greek Chicken Gyros

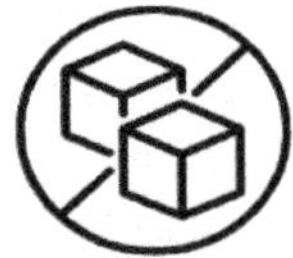
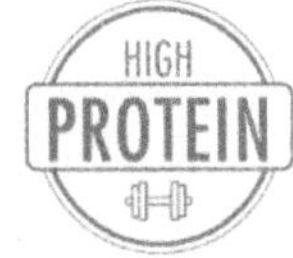

This recipe makes 4 servings

Ingredients

- 2 lbs. chicken breast strips
- 1/4 cup olive oil
- 1/4 cup non-fat Greek yogurt
- 1 Tbsp. Greek seasoning
- Pinch of salt and pepper
- 2 Tbsp. red wine vinegar
- 1 lemon zest and juice
- 4 pieces of gyro bread
- Crumbled feta cheese
- Sliced up veggies of your choice

Directions

1.) In a bowl, combine olive oil, Greek yogurt, Greek seasoning, salt, pepper, red wine vinegar, and juice and zest of the lemon. Set aside.

2.) Pour mixture over chicken in a freezer bag and let marinate in the refrigerator for at least 2 hours. Once you are ready to grill, take chicken out of fridge to sit at room temperature for about 15 minutes.

3.) Put grill on medium heat, place chicken onto grill, and cook for 5 minutes. Flip chicken and cook for another 5 minutes. Once chicken is cooked, then place in a pan with foil over it.

4.) Toast your gyro bread and then assemble your gyros with your choice of vegetables and feta cheese.

Greek Yogurt Parfait

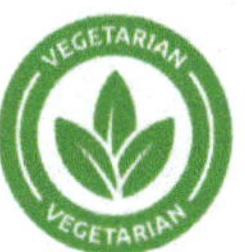

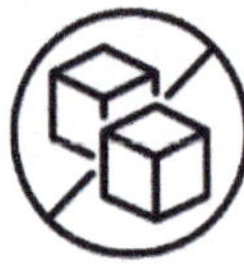
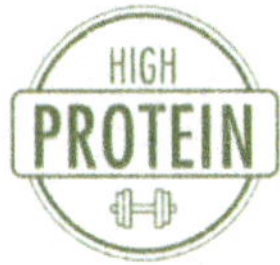

This recipe makes 1 serving

Ingredients

- 1 cup low-fat, low-sugar Greek yogurt
- 1/4 cup frozen or fresh mixed berries
- 2 Tbsp. low-sugar granola

Directions

1. Pour granola and some berries onto the bottom of a glass or bowl.
2. Scoop the yogurt on top of the granola.
3. Top the bowl with the remaining berries and sprinkle granola on the top.

Herbal Tea and Almond Oat Cookies

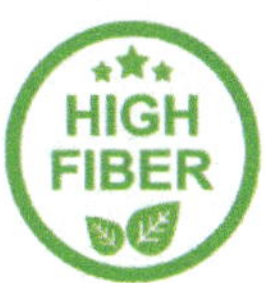

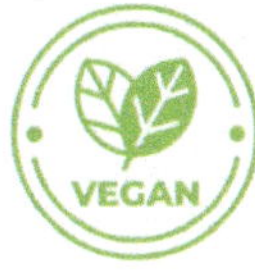

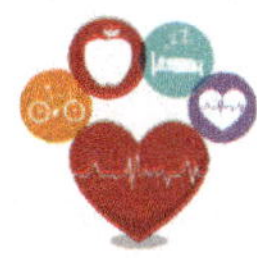
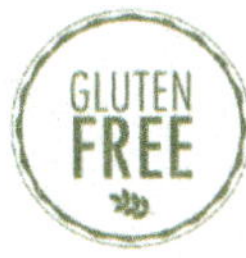

Serves 6

Ingredients

- 1 cup rolled gluten-free oats
- 1/2 cup almond flour
- 1/4 cup coconut oil, melted
- 1/4 cup maple syrup
- 1 tsp. vanilla extract
- 1/4 tsp. almond extract
- Pinch of salt
- Herbal tea for serving

Directions

1. Preheat the oven to 350 degrees F.
2. In a bowl, mix rolled oats, almond flour, melted coconut oil, maple syrup, vanilla extract, almond extract, and a pinch of salt.
3. Form small cookies and place them on a baking sheet.
4. Bake for 10-12 minutes, or until golden.
5. Serve with a cup of herbal tea. Chamomile, lavender, and lemon balm are particularly relaxing.

Kimchi Fried Rice

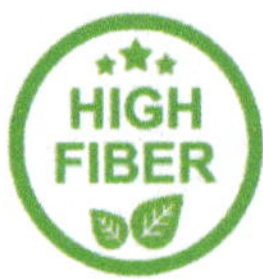

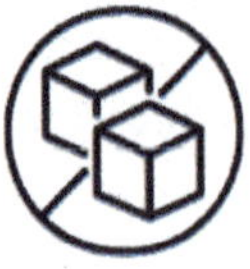

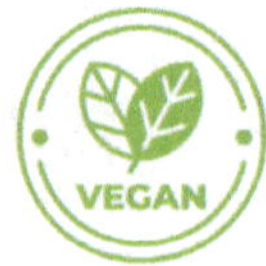

Serves 4

Ingredients

- 2 cups cooked brown rice
- 1 cup kimchi, chopped
- 1 cup mixed vegetables (carrots, peas, corn)
- 2 eggs, beaten
- 2 Tbsp. soy sauce
- 1 Tbsp. sesame oil
- Green onions for garnish

Directions

1. In a pan, sauté kimchi and mixed vegetables.
2. Add cooked rice and stir-fry.
3. Push the rice to one side and scramble the eggs on the other side.
4. Mix everything together and add soy sauce and sesame oil.
5. Garnish with green onions and serve.

Lentil and Tomato Stew with Kale

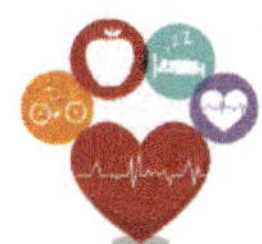
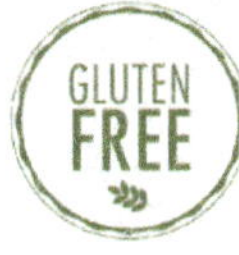

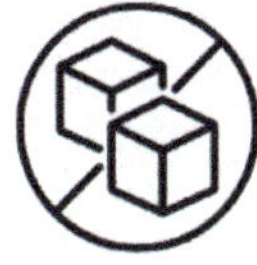
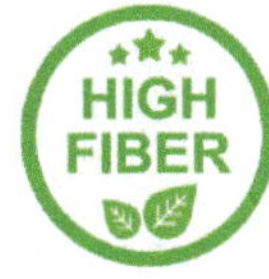

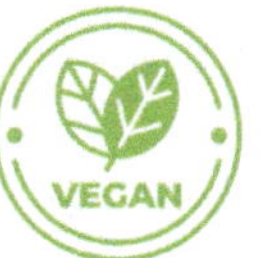

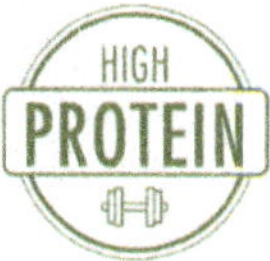

This recipe makes 4 servings

Ingredients

- 1 cup dried green lentils, rinsed
- 1 14 oz. can diced tomatoes
- 1 onion, chopped
- 3 cloves garlic, minced
- 1 tsp. cumin
- 1 tsp. smoked paprika
- 4 cups vegetable broth
- 2 cups kale, chopped
- Salt and pepper to taste

Directions

1. In a large pot, sauté the onion and garlic until softened.
2. Add lentil, diced tomatoes, cumin, smoked paprika, and vegetable broth.
3. Bring to a boil, then reduce heat and simmer for about 25-30 minutes, or until lentils are tender.
4. Stir in chopped kale and cook until wilted.
5. Season with salt and pepper to taste.

Make-Your-Own Trail Mix

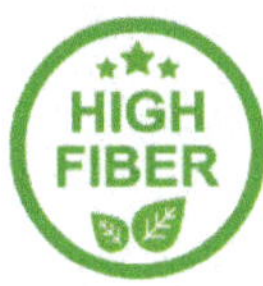

This recipe makes 10 servings

Ingredients

- 1/2 cup dried or freeze-dried fruit (cranberries, banana chips, mango slices, raisins, crystallized ginger, pineapple, apple, papaya, etc.)
- 1/2 cup nuts and seeds (unsalted roasted peanuts, unsalted cashews, unsalted sunflower seeds, unsalted roasted almonds, soy nuts, raw walnuts)
- 1 cup crunchy grains (low sugar granola, crispy whole grain cereal, pretzels, sesame sticks)
- 1/2 cup fun mix-ins (chocolate chips, yogurt covered raisins, chocolate covered raisins, shredded unsweetened coconut, mini-marshmallow.

Directions

1. Combine all ingredients together.
2. Store in an air-tight container and serve in small single-serving zip-top bags.

One Pot Taco Stew

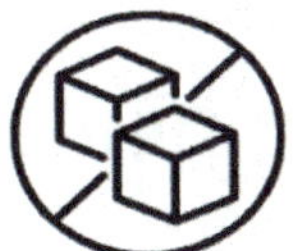

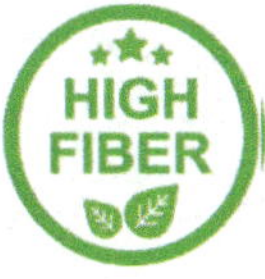

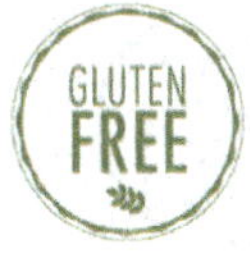

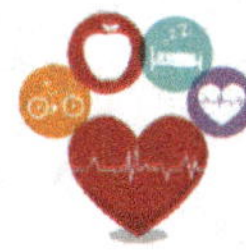

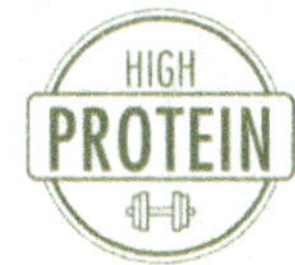

This recipe makes 6-8 servings

Ingredients

- 1 lb. lean ground turkey
- 2 cans black beans
- 1 can corn
- 2 cans diced tomatoes
- 1 onion, diced
- 1 can tomato sauce
- 2 tsp. chili powder
- 1 tsp. cumin
- Crushed tortilla chips
- Sour cream

Directions

1. Add oil to a pot. Over medium heat, brown ground turkey until no longer pink.
2. Drain black beans and corn. Add to turkey with diced tomatoes, onion, tomato sauce, and spices.
3. Lower heat and let cook until heated through.
4. Serve warm with crushed tortilla chips and sour cream.

Quinoa and Black Bean Salad

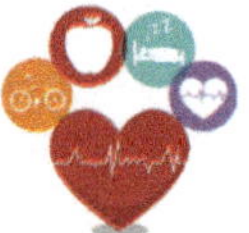
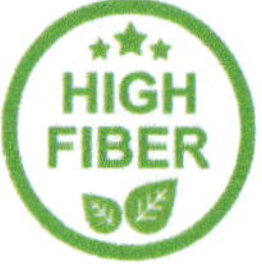

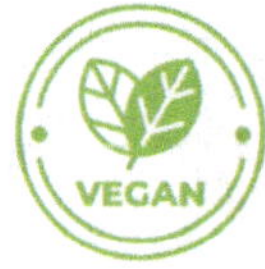

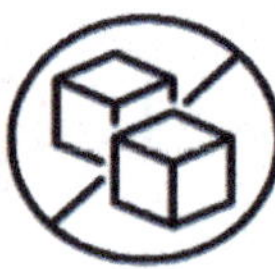
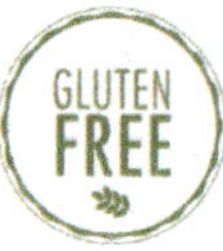

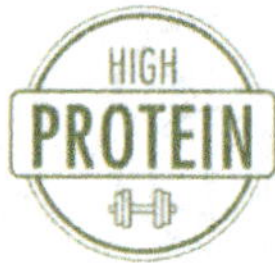

This recipe makes 4 servings

Ingredients

- 1 cup quinoa, rinsed and drained
- 1 15 oz. can low-sodium black beans, drained and rinsed
- 1 cup corn kernels (fresh, frozen, or canned)
- 1 red bell pepper, diced
- 1/4 cup chopped fresh cilantro
- Juice of 2 limes
- 2 Tbsp. olive oil
- Salt-free seasoning blend (to taste)

Directions

1. Cook quinoa according to package instructions and let it cool.
2. In a large bowl, combine quinoa, black beans, corn, red bell pepper, and cilantro.
3. In a separate bowl, whisk together lime juice and olive oil, then pour over the salad.
4. Season with salt-free seasoning blend and toss to combine.

Salmon and Avocado Sushi Bowl

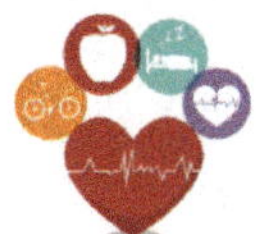
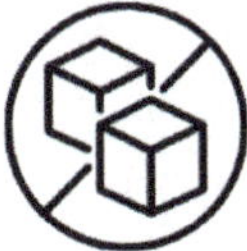
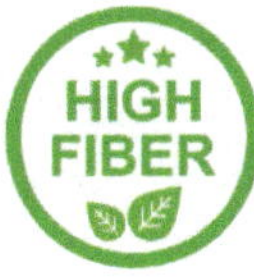

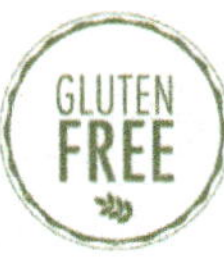

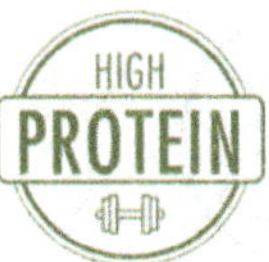

This recipe makes 2 servings

Ingredients

- 1 cup cooked brown rice
- 4 oz. grilled salmon, flaked
- 1/2 avocado, sliced
- 1/2 cucumber, sliced
- 1 Tbsp. soy sauce
- 1 tsp. sesame oil
- Seaweed flakes for garnish

Directions

1. Arrange brown rice in a bowl.
2. Top with grilled salmon, avocado, and cucumber.
3. Drizzle with soy sauce and sesame oil.
4. Garnish with seaweed flakes.
5. Mix ingredients and enjoy!

Tuna Patties

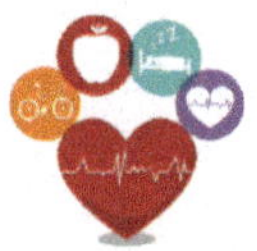
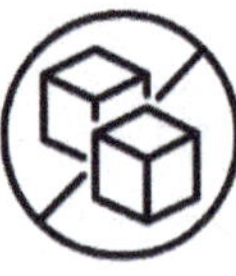
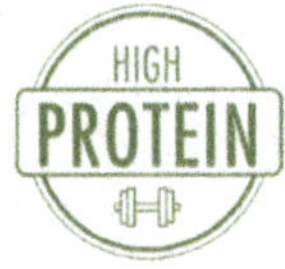

This recipe makes 2 servings

Ingredients

- 1 can light tuna in water
- 1 Tbsp. light mayo
- 1 Tbsp. plain Greek yogurt
- 1 egg
- 1 tsp. parsley flakes
- 1/4 yellow onion, diced
- 1/4 cup breadcrumbs
- 1 Tbsp. Dijon mustard
- 1 Tbsp. olive oil

Directions

1. Drain can of tuna. In medium bowl, mix together tuna, mayo, yogurt, egg, parsley, onion, breadcrumbs, and Dijon mustard.
2. Heat a pan with olive oil over medium heat.
3. Form patties and place on hot pan.
4. Cook until browned, and then flip.
5. Serve hot.

White Wine Risotto & Salmon

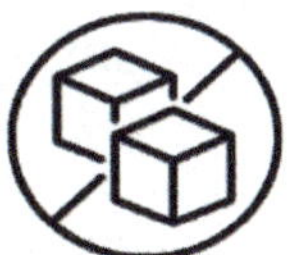
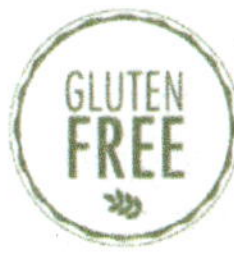

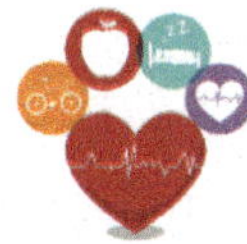
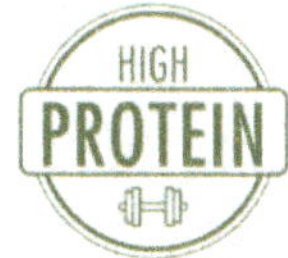

This recipe makes 6 servings

Tip: Making risotto is a very mindful practice, continually adding broth and mixing until you get the perfect consistency.

Ingredients

- 4 ¼ cup Arborio rice, dry
- 1.5 cups small white onions, diced
- 2 garlic cloves, minced
- 1 package fresh asparagus, chopped
- 6 baby portobello mushrooms, sliced
- 5 sun-dried tomatoes, chopped
- 2.5 cups vegetable broth
- 3 Tbsp. plain Greek yogurt
- 1 ¼ cup parmesan, shredded
- 1 cup white wine
- 1 fillet wild salmon
- 1/4 fennel bulb, diced
- 2 sprigs fresh dill, chopped
- 1/4 oz. Mirin
- 1 Tbsp. olive oil

Directions

1. Preheat oven to 350 degrees F
2. Place fish on top of parchment paper and cover with all seasonings, distributed evenly.
3. Cover with parchment paper. Fold all sides in so there are no openings. Cook for 18 minutes.
4. In a small pan, mix onion, garlic, and fennel in olive oil on medium-high heat for approximately 2 minutes.
5. Add mushrooms, rice, asparagus, mirin, and white wine to the pan. Let deglaze until all liquid is gone.
6. Add 1 cup vegetable broth. Stir occasionally, while gradually adding remaining vegetable stock until all rice is absorbed.
7. Once liquid is almost gone, add cheese and yogurt and vigorously stir until texture is creamy, not sticky. Add sun-dried tomatoes and enjoy!

APPENDIX A:

Hydration Tests

There are two ways I suggest testing to see if you are hydrated:

1.) The first test is examining the color of your urine. It should be as close to clear as possible. If it is dark colored, chances are you are dehydrated.
2.) The other test is to pinch the top of your hand. If the skin immediately returns to the hand, you are likely hydrated. If it takes more than a couple seconds, you are probably dehydrated.

APPENDIX B: ESSENTIAL NUTRIENTS FOR VEGANS

A vegan diet can offer numerous health benefits, but it's essential to be mindful of certain nutrients that may be lacking or present in lower quantities compared to omnivorous diets. While a well-planned vegan diet can provide all the necessary nutrients for optimal health, there are a few key vitamins, minerals, and nutrients that vegans should pay special attention to and consider supplementing if needed. These include vitamin B12, vitamin D, omega-3 fatty acids, iron, calcium, zinc, and iodine. Ensuring an adequate intake of these nutrients can help vegans maintain overall health and prevent deficiencies. Here's a breakdown of each:

Vitamin B12: Found primarily in animal products, vitamin B12 is crucial for nerve function and DNA synthesis. Vegans should consider fortified foods or supplements to meet their B12 needs.

Vitamin D: While vitamin D can be synthesized by the body through sunlight exposure, it may be challenging to obtain sufficient levels, especially in regions with limited sunlight. Fortified foods and supplements can help vegans meet their vitamin D requirements.

Omega-3 Fatty Acids: Sources of omega-3 fatty acids such as EPA and DHA are predominantly found in fish and seafood. Plant-based sources like flaxseeds, chia seeds, and walnuts provide ALA, a precursor to EPA and DHA, but supplementation may be necessary for some individuals to ensure adequate intake.

Iron: Plant-based sources of iron, such as lentils, beans, tofu, and spinach, are abundant, but the iron in these foods is less readily absorbed than heme iron from animal products. Consuming vitamin C-rich foods alongside iron-rich plant foods can enhance absorption.

Calcium: While dairy products are a traditional source of calcium, vegans can obtain this mineral from fortified plant milks, tofu, leafy greens like kale and collard greens, and calcium-set tofu. Calcium supplements may be warranted for those with low intakes or specific dietary restrictions.

Zinc: Plant-based sources of zinc include legumes, nuts, seeds, and whole grains. However, the phytates present in these foods can inhibit zinc absorption. To ensure adequate zinc intake, vegans may consider consuming zinc-rich foods regularly or using fortified foods or supplements.

Iodine: Iodine is primarily found in seafood and dairy products due to iodine supplementation in livestock feed. Vegans can obtain iodine from iodized salt and seaweed, but intake can vary. For those with limited iodine sources, iodine supplements or iodine-fortified foods may be beneficial.

By being mindful of these nutrients and incorporating fortified foods or supplements as needed, vegans can maintain a balanced and nutritious diet that supports their health and well-being.

Book Sponsor: Lifeway Kefir

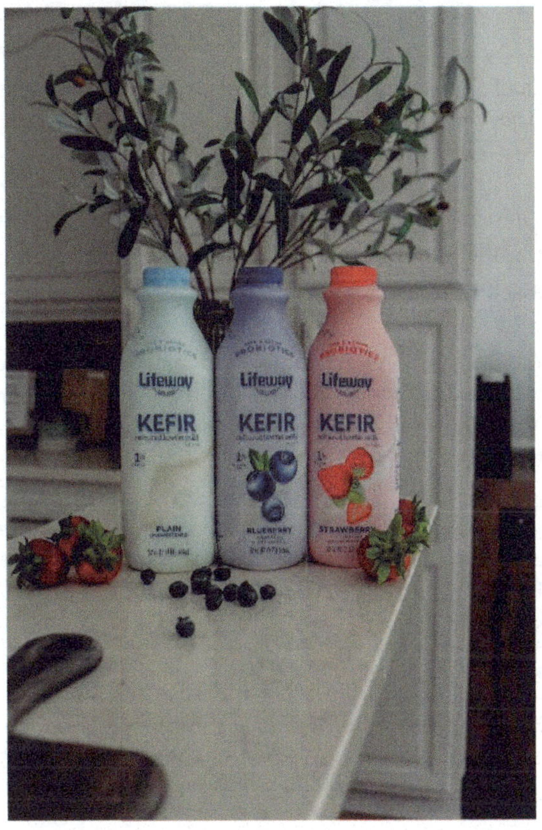

I am deeply grateful to Lifeway Kefir for their unwavering support and for being our book sponsor. Our decade-long partnership has been invaluable in spreading the message of health and wellness to families everywhere. Lifeway Kefir's commitment to producing high-quality products has been instrumental. With its nutritional profile packed with vitamin D, calcium, protein and probiotics, Lifeway Kefir stands as a convenient and delicious option for incorporating fermented foods into our diets, promoting gut health and overall well-being. Lifeway Kefir continues to lead the way in nurturing healthier lifestyles, and I am privileged to have them as a partner in our journey towards better health.

Visit Lifeway Kefir at lifewaykefir.com.

REFERENCES

[i] 6, Feb, and Jennifer Lubell. "In Age of GLP-1 Agonists, Food Choices Still Matter for Health." *American Medical Association*, 6 Feb. 2024, www.ama-assn.org/delivering-care/public-health/age-glp-1-agonists-food-choices-still-matter-health.

[ii] Chronic Diseases in America. Centers for Disease Control and Prevention. https://www.cdc.gov/chronicdisease/resources/infographic/chronic-diseases.htm. Published January 12, 2021. Accessed February 21, 2021.

[iii] Al-Maskari F. LIFESTYLE DISEASES: An Economic Burden on the Health Services. United Nations. https://www.un.org/en/chronicle/article/lifestyle-diseases-economic-burden-health-services#:~:text=Lifestyle%20diseases%20share%20risk%20factors,metabolic%20syndrome%2C%20chronic%20obstructive%20pulmonary. Accessed February 21, 2021.

[iv] Why Good Nutrition is Important. Center for Science in the Public Interest. https://www.cspinet.org/eating-healthy/why-good-nutrition-important#:~:text=Unhealthy%20eating%20and%20physical%20inactivity,cancer%2C%20and%20type%202%20diabetes. Published May 17, 2018. Accessed February 21, 2021.

[v] Tomas et al., "Mediterranean diet, cardiovascular disease and mortality in diabetes: A systematic review and meta-analysis of prospective cohort studies and randomized clinical trials" *Crit Rev Food Sci Nutr*. 2020;60(7):1207-1227. doi: 10.1080/10408398.2019.1565281. Epub 2019 Jan 24.

[vi] Gardener et al., "Effect of Low-Fat vs Low-Carbohydrate Diet on 12-Month Weight Loss in Overweight Adults and the Association with Genotype Pattern or Insulin SecretionThe DIETFITS Randomized Clinical Trial," JAMA, 2018;319(7):667-679. doi:10.1001.

[vii] Omar-Hmeadi, M., Lund, A., Seiron, P., Svensson, M. K., Krogvold, L., Dahl-Jørgensen, K., ... & Ahlqvist, E. (2020). Dysregulated glucagon secretion accompanies islet dysfunction in type 2 diabetes. *JCI Insight*, *5*(17), e139673.

[viiiviii] Mormon, M. John, "GLP-1 Medications and Weight Loss: Help Patients Navigate Beyond Trends." Wolters Kluwer, 19 July 2024, www.wolterskluwer.com/en/expert-insights/glp-1-medications-and-weight-loss-help-patients-navigate-beyond-trends. Accessed 29 July 2024.

[ix] Combining Medication and Nutrition Therapy for the Treatment of Type 2 Diabetes" (Diabetes Care, 2015).

[x] Fujiwara, Y., Eguchi, S., Murayama, H., Takahashi, Y., Toda, M., Imai, K., & Tsuda, K. (2019). Relationship between diet/exercise and pharmacotherapy to enhance the GLP-1 levels in type 2 diabetes. Endocrinology, Diabetes & Metabolism, 2(3), e00068. https://doi.org/10.1002/edm2.68

[xi] Van Ruiten, C. C., ten Kulve, J. S., van Bloemendaal, L., Nieuwdorp, M., Veltman, D. J., & IJzerman, R. G. (2022). Eating behavior modulates the sensitivity to the central effects of GLP-1 agonist receptor treatment: A secondary analysis of a randomized trial. *Psychoneuroendocrinology*, *137*, 105667. https://doi.org/10.1016/j.psyneuen.2022.105667

[xii] Watanabe, Y.; Saito, I.; Henmi, I.; Yoshimura, K.; Maruyama, K.; Yamauchi, K.; Matsuo, T.; Kato, T.; Tanigawa, T.; Kishida, T.; et al. Skipping Breakfast is Correlated with Obesity. J. *Rural Med*, 2014, 9, 51-58. [CrossRef] [PubMed].

[xiii] Bodnaruc, A. M., Prudhomme, D., Blanchet, R., and Giroux, I. (2016, December 9). *Nutritional modulation of endogenous glucagon-like peptide-1 secretion: A Review - Nutrition & Metabolism*. BioMed Central. https://nutritionandmetabolism.biomedcentral.com/articles/10.1186/s12986-016-0153-3

[xiv] de Munter JS, Hu FB, Spiegelman D, Franz M, van Dam RM, "Whole grain, bran, and germ intake and risk of type 2 diabetes: a prospective cohort study and systematic review," *PLoS Med*, 2007;4:e261.

[xv] Reynolds A, Mann J, Cummings J, Winter N, Mete E, Te Morenga L. "Carbohydrate quality and human health: a series of systematic reviews and meta-analyses," *Lancet,* 2019;393:434-45.

[xvi] Michaeleen Doucleff. "Less Snacking, More Satisfaction: Some Foods Boost Levels of an Ozempic-like Hormone." *NPR*, NPR, 30 Oct. 2023, www.npr.org/sections/health-shots/2023/10/30/1208883691/diet-ozempic-wegovy-weight-loss-fiber-glp-1-diabetes-barley.https://www.npr.org/sections/health-shots/2023/10/30/1208883691/diet-ozempic-wegovy-weight-loss-fiber-glp-1-diabetes-barley

[xvii] Harvard Health Publishing. (2024, February 5). Eat more fiber-rich foods to foster heart health. Reviewed by Howard E. LeWine, MD, Chief Medical Editor. Retrieved from https://www.health.harvard.edu/heart-health/eat-more-fiber-rich-foods-to-foster-heart-health#:~:text=Fiber's%20role%20in%20preventing%20heart,less%20and%20perhaps%20lose%20weight.

[xviii] Aune D, Norat T, Romundstad P, Vatten LJ, "Whole grain and refined grain consumption and the risk of type 2 diabetes: a systematic review and dose-response meta-analysis of cohort studies," *Eur J Epidemiol*, 2013;28:845-58.

[XIX] Ida, S., Kaneko, R., Imataka, K., Okubo, K., Shirakura, Y., Azuma, K., Fujiwara, R., & Murata, K. (2021). Effects of antidiabetic drugs on muscle mass in type 2 diabetes mellitus. *Current Diabetes Reviews*, *17*(3), 293–303. https://doi.org/10.2174/1573399816666200705210006

[xx] Sources and Amounts of Animal, Dairy, and Plant Protein Intake of US Adults in 2007-2010

[xxi] Stefan M. Pasiakos, Sanjiv Agarwal, Harris R. Lieberman, Victor L. Fulgoni, III

Nutrients. 2015 Aug; 7(8): 7058-7069. Published online 2015 Aug 21. doi: 10.3390/nu70853

[xxii] Howard, BV, Van Horn, L, Hsia, J, et al., "Low-fat dietary pattern and risk of cardiovascular disease: The Women's Health Initiative Randomized Controlled Dietary Modification Trial," *JAMA,* 2006; 295: 655-666.

[xxiii] Tobias, DK, Chen, M, Manson, JE, et al., "Effect of low-fat diet interventions versus other diet interventions on long-term weight change in adults: A systematic review and meta-analysis,"

Lancet Diabetes Endocrinol 2015; 3: 968-979.

[xxiv] Center for Food Safety and Applied Nutrition. "Trans Fat." *U.S. Food and Drug Administration*, 18 May 2018, www.fda.gov/food/food-additives-petitions/trans-fat.https://www.fda.gov/food/food-additives-petitions/trans-fat.

[xxv] American Heart Association. "Fish and Omega-3 Fatty Acids." *Www.heart.org*, 1 Nov. 2021, www.heart.org/en/healthy-living/healthy-eating/eat-smart/fats/fish-and-omega-3-fatty-acids. https://www.heart.org/en/healthy-living/healthy-eating/eat-smart/fats/fish-and-Omega-3-fatty-acids.

[xxvi] Simopoulos, Artemis. "An Increase in the Omega-6/Omega-3 Fatty Acid Ratio Increases the Risk for Obesity." *Nutrients*, vol. 8, no. 3, 2 Mar. 2016, p. 128, www.ncbi.nlm.nih.gov/pmc/articles/PMC4808858/.

[xxvii] Tutunchi H, Ostadrahimi A, Saghafi-Asl M. The Effects of Diets Enriched in Monounsaturated

Oleic Acid on the Management and Prevention of Obesity: a Systematic Review of Human

Intervention Studies. Adv Nutr. 2020 Jul 1;11(4):864-877. doi: 10.1093/advances/nmaa013. PMID: 32135008; PMCID: PMC7360458.

[xxviii] Blum, D. (2023, April 21). "An extreme risk of taking ozempic: Malnutrition." *The New York Times*. https://www.nytimes.com/2023/04/21/well/eat/ozempic-side-effects-malnutrition.html

[xxix] https://www.hsph.harvard.edu/nutritionsource/what-should-you-eat/vegetables-and-fruits/.

[xxx] Lee, Seung Hee. "Adults Meeting Fruit and Vegetable Intake Recommendations — United States, 2019." *MMWR. Morbidity and Mortality Weekly Report*, vol. 71, no. 1, 7 Jan. 2022, www.cdc.gov/mmwr/volumes/71/wr/mm7101a1.htm?s_cid=mm7101a1_w, https://doi.org/10.15585/mmwr.mm7101a1.https://www.cdc.gov/mmwr/volumes/71/wr/mm7101a1.htm?s_cid=mm7101a1_w.

[xxxi] "USDA ERS - a Closer Look at Declining Fruit and Vegetable Consumption Using Linked Data Sources." *Www.ers.usda.gov*, www.ers.usda.gov/amber-waves/2016/july/a-closer-look-at-declining-fruit-and-vegetable-consumption-using-linked-data-sources/. Accessed 23 July 2024.https://www.ers.usda.gov/amber-waves/2016/july/a-closer-look-at-declining-fruit-and-vegetable-consumption-using-linked-data-sources/.

[xxxii] Environmental Working Group. "Dirty Dozen™ Fruits and Vegetables with the Most Pesticides." *Ewg.org*, 2019, www.ewg.org/foodnews/dirty-dozen.php.https://www.ewg.org/foodnews/dirty-dozen.php.

[xxxiii] Winter CK, Katz JM. Dietary exposure to pesticide residues from commodities alleged to contain the highest contamination levels. *J Toxicol*. 2011;2011:589674. doi:10.1155/2011/589674

[xxxiv] Prior, R. L., et al. "Analysis of Botanicals and Dietary Supplements for Antioxidant Capacity: A Review." *Journal of AOAC International*, vol. 83, no. 4, 1 July 2000, pp. 950–956, pubmed.ncbi.nlm.nih.gov/10995120/. https://pubmed.ncbi.nlm.nih.gov/10995120/

[xxxv] Wolfe, Kelly L., et al. "Cellular Antioxidant Activity of Common Fruits." *Journal of Agricultural and Food Chemistry*, vol. 56, no. 18, 24 Sept. 2008, pp. 8418–8426, pubmed.ncbi.nlm.nih.gov/18759450/, https://doi.org/10.1021/jf801381y.https://pubs.acs.org/doi/abs/10.1021/jf801381y

[xxxvi] Ullah, Asad, et al. "Important Flavonoids and Their Role as a Therapeutic Agent." *Molecules*, vol. 25, no. 22, 11 Nov. 2020, p. 5243, https://doi.org/10.3390/molecules25225243.https://pubmed.ncbi.nlm.nih.gov/33187049/

[xxxvii] Arballo J, Amengual J, Erdman JW. Lycopene: A Critical Review of Digestion, Absorption, Metabolism, and Excretion. *Antioxidants*. 2021;10(3):342. doi:10.3390/antiox10030342.

[xxxviii] Abdul Hakim BN, Yahya HM, Shahar S, Abdul Manaf Z, Damanhuri H. Effect of Sequence of Fruit Intake in a Meal on Satiety. Int J Environ Res Public Health. 2019 Nov 13;16(22):4464. doi: 10.3390/ijerph16224464. PMID: 31766283; PMCID: PMC6888291.

[xxxix] airing carbs with fiber, and consuming sources consistently throughout the day, can help to stabilize your blood sugar levels and provide your body with sustainable energy throughout the day.

[xl] American Heart Association. "Fish and Omega-3 Fatty Acids." *Www.heart.org*, 1 Nov. 2021, www.heart.org/en/healthy-living/healthy-eating/eat-smart/fats/fish-and-omega-3-fatty-acids.

[xli] Dorton, H. M., Luo, S., Monterosso, J. R., & Page, K. A. (2018). Influences of dietary added sugar consumption on striatal food-cue reactivity and postprandial GLP-1 response. *Frontiers in Psychiatry, 8*. https://doi.org/10.3389/fpsyt.2017.00297

[xlii] Jones, S., Luo, S., Dorton, H. M., Yunker, A. G., Angelo, B., Defendis, A., Monterosso, J. R., & Page, K. A. (2021). Obesity and Dietary Added Sugar Interact to Affect Postprandial GLP-1 and Its Relationship to Striatal Responses to Food Cues and Feeding Behavior. Frontiers in Endocrinology, 12, 638504. https://doi.org/10.3389/fendo.2021.638504

[xliii] Artificial Sweeteners Negatively Regulate Pathogenic Characteristics of Two Model Gut Bacteria, *E. coli* and *E. faecalis*" by Aparna Shil and Havovi Chichger, 15 May 2021, *International Journal of Molecular Sciences*.

[xliv] Mathilde Touvier, PhD, director, nutritional epidemiology research team, French National Institute for Health and Medical Research and Sorbonne Paris Nord University, Bobigny, France; Charlotte Debras, PhD candidate, French National Institute for Health and Medical Research and Sorbonne Paris Nord University; Amy Bragagnini, MS, RD, oncology dietitian, Mercy Health Saint Mary's Campus, Lacks Cancer Center, Grand Rapids, Mich.; Marji McCullough, ScD, RD, senior scientific director, epidemiology research, American Cancer Society, Atlanta; Calorie Control Council, written statement, March 23, 2022; *PLOS Medicine*, March 24, 2022, online.

[xlv] Centers for Disease Control and Prevention. (n.d.). Sodium intake and health. Retrieved Marc 31, 2024 from https://www.cdc.gov/salt/index.htm

[xlvi] Huang, Liping, et al. "Effect of Dose and Duration of Reduction in Dietary Sodium on Blood Pressure Levels: Systematic Review and Meta-Analysis of Randomised Trials." *BMJ*, vol. 368, 24 Feb. 2020, p. m315,
https://doi.org/10.1136/bmj.m315.https://www.bmj.com/content/368/bmj.m315

[xlvii] CDC. "About Sodium and Health." *Salt*, 19 Apr. 2024, www.cdc.gov/salt/about/index.html.

[xlviii] Cahill Leah E, Chiuve Stephanie E, Mekary Rania A, Jensen Majken K, Flint Alan J, Hu Frank B, et al. Prospective study of breakfast eating and incident coronary heart disease in a cohort of male US health professionals. Circulation. 2013;128(4):337-43.

[xlix] Jakubowicz, Daniela, et al. "Fasting until Noon Triggers Increased Postprandial Hyperglycemia and Impaired Insulin Response after Lunch and Dinner in Individuals with Type 2 Diabetes: A Randomized Clinical Trial." *Diabetes Care*, vol. 38, no. 10, 2015, pp. 1820–6, www.ncbi.nlm.nih.gov/pubmed/26220945, https://doi.org/10.2337/dc15-0761.https://pubmed.ncbi.nlm.nih.gov/26220945/

[l] "High-Energy Breakfast Promotes Weight Loss." *EurekAlert!*, www.eurekalert.org/news-releases/559766. Accessed 23 July 2024. https://www.eurekalert.org/news-releases/559766

[li] Ghazzawi, H. A., & Mustafa, S. (2019). Effect of high-protein breakfast meal on within-day appetite hormones: Peptide YY, glucagon like peptide-1 in adults. *Clinical Nutrition Experimental*, 28, 111-122.

[lii] American College of Sports Medicine, American School Health Association, GENYOUth Foundation, National Dairy Council, *The Wellness Impact: Enhancing Academic Through Healthy School Environment,* March 2013.

[liii] Melore, Chris. "Breakfast Really Is for Champions: People Who Regularly Eat Morning Meal Happier, More Successful." *Study Finds*, 22 Mar. 2021, studyfinds.org/breakfast-for-champions-morning-meal-happier-more-successful/.https://studyfinds.org/breakfast-for-champions-morning-meal-happier-more-successful/

[liv] Pengpid, Supa, and Karl Peltzer. "Skipping Breakfast and Its Association with Health Risk Behaviour and Mental Health among University Students in 28 Countries." *Diabetes, Metabolic Syndrome and Obesity: Targets and Therapy*, vol. Volume 13, Aug. 2020, pp. 2889–2897, https://doi.org/10.2147/dmso.s241670.
https://www.ncbi.nlm.nih.gov/pmc/articles/PMC7443458/

[lv] Suni, Eric. "Sleep Statistics." *Sleep Foundation*, 26 Sept. 2023, www.sleepfoundation.org/how-sleep-works/sleep-facts-statistics.

[lvi] St-Onge, Marie-Pierre, et al. "Fiber and Saturated Fat Are Associated with Sleep Arousals and Slow Wave Sleep." *Journal of Clinical Sleep Medicine*, vol. 12, no. 01, 15 Jan. 2016, pp. 19–24, jcsm.aasm.org/viewabstract.aspx?pid=30412, https://doi.org/10.5664/jcsm.5384. Accessed 8 July 2019.

Fiber and Saturated Fat Are Associated with Sleep Arousals and Slow Wave Sleep - PubMed (nih.gov)

[lvii] Reutrakul S, Sumritsopak R, Saetung S, Chanprasertyothin S, Anothaisintawee T. The relationship between sleep and glucagon-like peptide 1 in patients with abnormal glucose tolerance. J Sleep Res. 2017 Dec;26(6):756-763. doi: 10.1111/jsr.12552. Epub 2017 May 31. PMID: 28560837.

[lviii] Suni, Eric, and Abhinav Singh. "Technology in the Bedroom." *Sleep Foundation*, 18 Apr. 2022, www.sleepfoundation.org/bedroom-environment/technology-in-the-bedroom#:~:text=Using%20devices%20tends%20to%20delay.

[lix] St-Onge, Marie-Pierre, et al. "Fiber and Saturated Fat Are Associated with Sleep Arousals and Slow Wave Sleep." *Journal of Clinical Sleep Medicine*, vol. 12, no. 01, 15 Jan. 2016, pp. 19–24, jcsm.aasm.org/viewabstract.aspx?pid=30412, https://doi.org/10.5664/jcsm.5384.

[lx] Andrews, Linda. "Journaling before Bed Can Help You Sleep." *Healthgrades*, 12 Nov. 2014, www.healthgrades.com/right-care/sleep-disorders/journaling-before-bed-can-help-ward-off-sleeplessness.

[lxi] Scullin, Michael K., et al. "The Effects of Bedtime Writing on Difficulty Falling Asleep: A Polysomnographic Study Comparing To-Do Lists and Completed Activity Lists." *Journal of Experimental Psychology: General*, vol. 147, no. 1, 1 Jan. 2018, pp. 139–146, pubmed.ncbi.nlm.nih.gov/29058942/, https://doi.org/10.1037/xge0000374.

[lxii] "People at Risk of Hoarding Disorder May Have Serious Complaints about Sleep." *EurekAlert!*, www.eurekalert.org/news-releases/612155.

[lxiii] Johns Hopkins Medicine. "The Dangers of Uncontrolled Sleep Apnea." *Johns Hopkins Medicine*, 2020, www.hopkinsmedicine.org/health/wellness-and-prevention/the-dangers-of-uncontrolled-sleep-apnea.

[lxiv] Coppola D. Annual sales of retail food and beverages in the United States from 1992 to 2019. Statistica website. https://www.statista.com/statistics/197619/annual-food-and-beverage-store-sales-in-the-us-since-1992/#:~:text=Annual%20sales%20of%20retail%20food,in%20the%20U.S.%201992%2D2019&text=This%20statistic%20shows%20the%20annual,approximately%20765.06%20billion%20U.S.%20dollars. Published November 30, 2020. Accessed June 16, 2021.

[lxv] USDA, Economic Research Service. America's Eating Habits: Food Away from Home. USDA website. https://www.ers.usda.gov/webdocs/publications/90228/eib-196_ch7.pdf?v=8116.5. Accessed June 16, 2021.

[lxvi] Du Y, Rong S, Sun Y, et al. Association between frequency of eating away-from-home meals and risk of all-cause and cause-specific mortality. *J Acad Nutr Diet.* 2021;121(9):1741-1749.e1. doi:10.1016/j.jand.2021.01.012

[lxvii] McCrory, Megan A., et al. "Fast-Food Offerings in the United States in 1986, 1991, and 2016 Show Large Increases in Food Variety, Portion Size, Dietary Energy, and Selected Micronutrients." *Journal of the Academy of Nutrition and Dietetics*, vol. 119, no. 6, Feb. 2019, www.sciencedirect.com/science/article/pii/S2212267218323839, https://doi.org/10.1016/j.jand.2018.12.004.

[lxviii] Hollands, Gareth J, et al. "Portion, Package or Tableware Size for Changing Selection and Consumption of Food, Alcohol and Tobacco." *Cochrane Database of Systematic Reviews*, no. 9, 14 Sept. 2015, https://doi.org/10.1002/14651858.cd011045.pub2.

[lxix] Staff, Review. "Cornell Bottomless Soup Bowl Experiment." *The Cornell Review*, 12 June 2010, www.thecornellreview.org/cornell-bottomless-soup-bowl-experiment/.

[lxx] Burmeister, Jacob M., and Robert A. Carels. "Television Use and Binge Eating in Adults Seeking Weight Loss Treatment." *Eating Behaviors*, vol. 15, no. 1, Jan. 2014, pp. 83–86, https://doi.org/10.1016/j.eatbeh.2013.10.001.

[lxxi] Biddle, Stuart J.H., et al. "Screen Time, Other Sedentary Behaviours, and Obesity Risk in Adults: A Review of Reviews." *Current Obesity Reports*, vol. 6, no. 2, 1 June 2017, pp. 134–147, link.springer.com/article/10.1007%2Fs13679-017-0256-9, https://doi.org/10.1007/s13679-017-0256-9. Accessed 24 June 2020. Screen Time, Other Sedentary Behaviours, and Obesity Risk in Adults: A Review of Reviews—PubMed (nih.gov)

[lxxii] "Mindful Eating." *The Nutrition Source*, 14 Sept. 2020, nutritionsource.hsph.harvard.edu/mindful-eating/. Mindful Eating | The Nutrition Source | Harvard T.H. Chan School of Public Health

[lxxiii] Pegah, A., Abbasi-Oshaghi, E., Khodadadi, I., Mirzaei, F., & Tayebinaia, H. (2021). Probiotic and resveratrol normalize GLP-1 levels and oxidative stress in the intestine of diabetic rats. Metabol Open, 10, 100093. https://doi.org/10.1016/j.metop.2021.100093

[lxxiv] Rahman, Md. Mominur, et al. "The Gut Microbiota (Microbiome) in Cardiovascular Disease and Its Therapeutic Regulation." *Frontiers in Cellular and Infection Microbiology*, vol. 12, 20 June 2022, https://doi.org/10.3389/fcimb.2022.903570.

[lxxv] https://www.heart.org/en/news/2018/05/01/gut-bacteria-may-impact-body-weight-fat-and-good-cholesterol-levels

[lxxvi]Madison, Annelise, and Janice K Kiecolt-Glaser. "Stress, Depression, Diet, and the Gut Microbiota: Human–Bacteria Interactions at the Core of Psychoneuroimmunology and Nutrition." *Current Opinion in Behavioral Sciences*, vol. 28, no. 3, Aug. 2019, pp. 105–110, www.sciencedirect.com/science/article/pii/S2352154618301608, https://doi.org/10.1016/j.cobeha.2019.01.011.

[lxxvii] Clarke, Gerard, et al. "Minireview: Gut Microbiota: The Neglected Endocrine Organ." *Molecular Endocrinology*, vol. 28, no. 8, Aug. 2014, pp. 1221–1238, www.ncbi.nlm.nih.gov/pmc/articles/PMC5414803/, https://doi.org/10.1210/me.2014-1108.

[lxxviii] Han, Hui, et al. "From Gut Microbiota to Host Appetite: Gut Microbiota-Derived Metabolites as Key Regulators." *Microbiome*, vol. 9, no. 1, 20 July 2021, microbiomejournal.biomedcentral.com/articles/10.1186/s40168-021-01093-y, https://doi.org/10.1186/s40168-021-01093-y.

[lxxix] Siddiqui, Ruqaiyyah, et al. "The Gut Microbiome and Female Health." *Biology*, vol. 11, no. 11, 1 Nov. 2022, p. 1683, www.mdpi.com/2079-7737/11/11/1683, https://doi.org/10.3390/biology11111683.

[lxxx] Zheng, Danping, et al. "Interaction between Microbiota and Immunity in Health and Disease." *Cell Research*, vol. 30, no. 6, 20 May 2020, pp. 492–506, https://doi.org/10.1038/s41422-020-0332-7.

[lxxxi] https://www.heart.org/en/news/2018/05/01/gut-bacteria-may-impact-body-weight-fat-and-good-cholesterol-levels

[lxxxii] Wu, Hsin-Jung, and Eric Wu. "The Role of Gut Microbiota in Immune Homeostasis and Autoimmunity." *Gut Microbes*, vol. 3, no. 1, 1 Jan. 2012, pp. 4–14, www.ncbi.nlm.nih.gov/pmc/articles/PMC3337124/, https://doi.org/10.4161/gmic.19320.

[lxxxiii] Reynolds, Andrew, et al. "Carbohydrate Quality and Human Health: A Series of Systematic Reviews and Meta-Analyses." *The Lancet*, vol. 393, no. 10170, Feb. 2019, pp. 434–445, https://doi.org/10.1016/s0140-6736(18)31809-9.

[lxxxiv] Frame, Leigh A, et al. "Current Explorations of Nutrition and the Gut Microbiome: A Comprehensive Evaluation of the Review Literature." *Nutrition Reviews*, vol. 78, no. 10, 25 Mar. 2020, pp. 798–812, https://doi.org/10.1093/nutrit/nuz106.

[lxxxv] Vij, Vinu Ashok Kumar, and Anjali S. Joshi. "Effect of Excessive Water Intake on Body Weight, Body Mass Index, Body Fat, and Appetite of Overweight Female Participants." *Journal of Natural Science, Biology, and Medicine*, vol. 5, no. 2, 2014, pp. 340–344, www.ncbi.nlm.nih.gov/pmc/articles/PMC4121911/, https://doi.org/10.4103/0976-9668.136180.

[lxxxvii] Thornton, Simon N. "Increased Hydration Can Be Associated with Weight Loss." *Frontiers in Nutrition*, vol. 3, no. 18, 10 June 2016, www.ncbi.nlm.nih.gov/pmc/articles/PMC4901052/, https://doi.org/10.3389/fnut.2016.00018.

[lxxxviii] Cooney, Olivia D., et al. "Healthy Gut, Healthy Bones: Targeting the Gut Microbiome to Promote Bone Health." *Frontiers in Endocrinology*, vol. 11, 19 Feb. 2021, https://doi.org/10.3389/fendo.2020.620466. Accessed 1 Mar. 2021. https://www.ncbi.nlm.nih.gov/pmc/articles/PMC7933548/#:~:text=Recently%2C%20the%20gut%20microbiome%20has,those%20with%20osteopenia%20or%20osteoporosis.

Made in United States
North Haven, CT
06 May 2025